Quick Medical Terminology:

A Self-Teaching Guide

4th Edition

Shirley Soltesz Steiner, R.N., M.S.

John Wiley & Sons, Inc.

Wiley also publishes its books in a variety of electronic formats. Some content that appears in
print may not be available in electronic books. For more information about Wiley products,
visit our web site at www.wiley.com.

ISBN 0-471-23359-5

Printed in the United States of America

10 9 8 7 6 5

For

Dorothy Elizabeth Wilson Soltesz who is my mom and best friend.

Mildred Hall who is my godmother and may not know how much she influenced my growing up years. Mildred assured me I had what it takes to go to college, get an education, and create a better life.

Contents

To the Reader

What It Is and Who It's For

So you want to learn the language of medicine. Great! Everything you need for learning medical terminology is right in your hands. The language of medicine is precise and technically oriented. It is among the great tools of the mind for better understanding and more accurate communication between all practitioners of the life sciences. Learning this special language is your opportunity to be among them. *Quick Medical Terminology* can prepare you for a new job or even a new career in one of the nation's fastest growing job markets, Health Care and Allied Health Services.

In *Quick Medical Terminology* you'll learn to pronounce, spell, and define medical terms used in today's health care settings. You will use a word-building strategy that helps you discover connections and relationships among word roots, prefixes, and suffixes. You'll learn the meaning of each part of a complex medical term and be able to put the parts together and define the term. Very quickly you'll develop a large repertoire of useful medical terms, much greater than the 500-plus terms presented in this text.

Quick Medical Terminology is an enjoyable way to learn the very special language of medicine by yourself, at your own pace. If you speak and understand English and have a high school education or equivalent, you'll quickly learn the basics and much more.

How to Use This Program

We suggest you use the following steps to approach your learning.

Step 1. Pre- and Post-Testing

If it's worth learning, isn't it worth knowing you have succeeded? You will find two Final Self-Tests in the back of your guide. We suggest you take one test before you begin your study and take another after you have completed all your lessons. Pre- and post-testing shows you how much you have learned. Either one of the final tests may be used first.

Step 2. Self-Instructional Unit

This self-teaching guide lets you proceed at a pace that is right for you. It provides everything you need to complete each of the ten instructional units, which include:

Introduction and Mini-Glossary.   The first page of each unit introduces you to what you will cover and provides a Mini-Glossary of the terms and word parts you'll be learning. You may want to refer to it as you proceed through the lesson.

Numbered frames.   Numbered frames are the building blocks of each unit. A frame presents a small amount of information and expects you to read and think about that information. Then it asks you to respond to it.

The way you respond may be:

- to select a medical term or definition from a list of suggested answers.

- to write a medical term for a given definition.

- to draw a conclusion and write it in your own words.

Example
Emesis is a term that means vomiting. A term that means excessive vomiting is *hyperemesis.* Underline the part of the medical term meaning excessive.

> A gallbladder attack can cause excessive vomiting. Write the term that describes this unpleasant condition. _____

Example
Myelo / dysplasia means defective development of the spinal cord.

> *Chondro* means cartilage. What does chondro / dysplasia mean? _____

Answers.   As you work through the unit, you'll find the correct answers on the left-hand side of the page. It's a good idea to use a folded piece of paper to cover the answer until you give your own. Your answer will be correct most of the time, but when your answer doesn't match ours, be sure you know why it doesn't. You may need to go back and review a few frames before continuing.

Pronunciation Guide.   When you work with a medical term for the first time, the answer column guides your pronunciation of the new term. Take the opportunity to practice pronouncing each new term correctly several times. Say it aloud or subverbally (saying it to yourself).

Example
chondrodysplasia (kon'dro dis pla'zhe)

Review Exercises.   Some units are longer than others, so to help you plan your breaks, we designed several short learning sequences into each unit. A brief

Review Exercise occurs at the end of a learning sequence. If you need a break, stop after a Review Exercise. Proceed at a pace that is right for you. We urge you to complete an entire unit before calling it a day.

Summary Exercise.   Each of the ten instructional units ends with a Summary Exercise. This final exercise pulls together all the new terms you worked with in the unit. Using the pronunciation guide alongside each term in the list, take the opportunity to practice pronouncing each term correctly and defining it aloud or subverbally. It really works! You might ask a friend to pronounce each term in the list so you can practice spelling it when you hear it.
[This is a good classroom exercise for instructor-guided spelling practice, pronunciation practice and defining the terms.]

Unit Self-Test.   Each unit ends with a Self-Test in two parts. Part 1 asks you to match a list of definitions with the correct medical terms. Part 2 asks you to construct the correct medical term for each definition listed. All terms and definitions are covered in the instructional unit you have just completed. Here's another opportunity to see how you're doing.

Step 3. Unit Review Sheet

Beginning on page 247, you'll find a two-part Review Sheet for each of the ten units of instruction that make up this self-teaching program. We suggest you begin every new unit (beginning with Unit 2) by completing a Review Sheet for the previous unit. These exercises are an important part of the learning program and will help you recall and practice the terms and definitions of the preceding unit before you begin the next one.

Part 1: Given a term, or word part, write the meaning.

Part 2: Given the definition of a term, write the correct term.

Correct answers are provided.

You may use these Review Sheets anytime, and as often as you wish. We suggest you make several photocopies of each Review Sheet and use them at any time to practice what you've already covered. There is never enough practice.

Objectives of the Program

When you have finished *Quick Medical Terminology,* you will have formed well over 500 medical terms using our word–building strategy combining prefixes, suffixes, and word roots to create complex medical terms.

1. You will learn to understand medical terms by breaking them into their component parts and learning the meaning of the parts.

2. You will learn to construct medical terms from component parts to express given definitions.

3. You will learn to pronounce, spell, and define medical terms used in this book.

4. You will be able to apply this word–building strategy to terms covered in this book and others you will come across as you work in a health care setting.

Pronunciation Key

The primary stress mark (′) is placed after the syllable bearing the heavier stress or accent; the secondary stress mark (′) follows a syllable having a somewhat lighter stress, as in *com·men·da·tion* (kom′ ən·dā′ shən).

a	add, map	m	move, seem	u	up, done
ā	ace, rate	n	nice, tin	er	urn, term
air	care, air	ng	ring, song	yo͞o	use, few
ä	palm, father	o	odd, hot	v	vain, eve
b	bat, rub	ō	open, so	w	win, away
ch	check, catch	ô	order, jaw	y	yet, yearn
d	dog, rod	oi	oil, boy	z	zest, muse
e	end, pet	ou	out, now	zh	vision, pleasure
ē	even, tree	o͞o	pool, food	ə	the schwa, an
f	fit, half	oo	took, full		unstressed vowel
g	go, log	p	pit, stop		representing the
h	hope, hate	r	run, poor		sound spelled
i	it, give	s	see, pass		*a* in *above*
ī	ice, write	sh	sure, rush		*e* in *sicken*
j	joy, ledge	t	talk, sit		*i* in *clarity*
k	cool, take	th	thin, both		*o* in *melon*
l	look, rule	th	this, bathe		*u* in *focus*

Source: Slightly modified "Pronunciation Key" in *Funk & Wagnalls Standard College Dictionary.* Copyright © 1977 by Harper & Row, Publishers, Inc. Reprinted by permission of the publisher.

The schwa (ə) varies widely in quality from a sound close to the (u) in *up* to a sound close to the (i) in *it* as heard in pronunciations of such words as *ballot, custom, landed, horses.*

The (r) in final position as in *star* (stär) and before a consonant as in *heart* (härt) is regularly indicated in the respellings, but pronunciations without (r) are unquestionably reputable. Standard British is much like the speech of Eastern New England and the Lower South in this feature.

In a few words, such as *button* (but′n) and *sudden* (sud′n), no vowel appears in the unstressed syllable because the (n) constitutes the whole syllable.

The Word-Building Strategy

Quick Medical Terminology teaches you a strategy for word-building. The vocabulary of medicine is large and complex, but you can learn much of it by breaking down a complex term into its meaningful parts and putting together a word from those meaningful parts. Let's begin.

1.
All words have a word root. The *root* is the base or the foundation of the word, regardless of what other word, unit, or syllable may be attached to it.

For example: *do* is the root of un*do* and *do*ing.

What is the root of import, export, transport, and support?

port _____

2.
In this example, the words suffix, prefix, affix, and fixation have fix

root as their _____.

3.
What is the root in tonsill/itis, tonsill/ectomy, and tonsill/ar?

tonsil _____.

4.
Two or more words may be combined to form a meaningful compound word. Using two or more of the following words, create some meaningful compound words:

Some Suggestions: over   stand
overhang   hang   wear
overcome   under   come
understand   grand   out
grandstand
outcome,   _____
etc.   _____
                           _____

5.

yes

two words are
   combined to make
   a meaningful
   compound term

Is teaspoon a compound word? _____

Explain your answer.

_____

_____

6.

A word root and a whole word may form a compound word. But
the root must be in its *combining form*. The root plus a vowel (a, e, i,
o, u) makes the combining form. Here are two compound terms,
micr/o/scope and tel/e/cast.

micr
tel

What are the word roots? _____;

micr/o
tel/e

What are the combining forms?_____.

7.

phon/ograph
gastr/o/enteric
laryng/o/spasm

Underline the combining form in each of the following words:

phon/o/graph   gastr/o/enter/ic
laryng/o/spasm

8.

a word root plus
   a vowel (a, e, i, o, u)

The combining form in compound words is made up of a
_____ plus a _____.

9.

In tel/e/graph and tel/e/phone the root plus a vowel is necessary to
make these compound words. What is this special form called?

a combining form

_____ _____.

10.

Compound terms may be composed of which of the following?
a) two or more whole words
b) a whole word and a word root
c) a word root combining form and a word

all three

Your answer? _____

11.

combining form

Two roots may join together but one of them will be in a special
form called the _____ _____.

12.

What kind of words are these: microfilm and telecommunication?

compound terms

_____

a combining form
(a root plus a vowel)
a whole word

What word parts are these terms made of? _____

_____

_____

13.

Many medical terms are made of a combining form, a word root, and an ending. In the term micr/o/scop/ic,

micr/o

the combining form is _____;

–ic

the ending is _____;

micr–

the root is _____;

Is there another word root? _____

scop–

What might it be? _____

14.

There are two word roots in micr/o/scop/ic. The root *micr* is in the combining form because it is attached to a word that begins with a consonant. There is no need to add a vowel to the root *scop* because

vowel

the ending -*ic* begins with a _____.

15.

Build a term from the combining form electr/o, the word root stat, and the ending -ic.

electrostatic

_____ / _____ / _____ / _____

16.

In the word hydroelectric,

word root

electr is the _____;

word

hydro is the _____;

ending

–ic is the _____.

17.

Endings change the basic meaning of a root or foundation word. Examine the following sentences:

    Joe's job was blast-ing the rocks.
    Tejo was blast-ed by the cannon.

ending

The meaning of *blast* is changed by its _____.

18.
A *suffix* is a word unit or syllable added to the end of a word or root that alters its meaning and creates a new word. In the words plant/er, plant/ed, and plant/ing, are these endings also suffixes? ___ Explain your answer.

yes
the endings added to the root changed its meaning

_____

_____.

19.
You can change the meaning of a word (or root) by adding a suffix. The suffix *-er* means *one who*. The word *port* means *to carry*. *Add* the suffix to the word root, *write* the word, and *explain* what it means.

porter
one who carries

_____   _____.

20.
When *-able* is added to the end of *read* it forms the new word *readable*. –Able is a meaningful unit added to the end of a word, creating a new word. So -able is a _____.

suffix

21.
A *prefix* is a meaningful unit joined to the beginning of a word or root that creates a new term. In the words im/plant, sup/plant, and trans/plant, the prefixes are _____, _____, and _____.

im-, sup-,
trans-

22.
In the word dis/please, *dis-* is a meaningful unit that comes before the word and changes the meaning of please; dis- is a _____.

prefix

23.
Meaningful units that go in front of a root are called prefixes. Meaningful units placed after a root are called suffixes.

Label the units in this word:

un-   manage   -able

prefix   *root*   *suffix*

_____   _____   _____

24.
A suffix or a prefix is called a meaningful unit because when it is attached or added to a root or word it changes the _____ of the _____.

meaning
word

our suggestion:

-itis is a word unit
added to the end of
a word altering its
meaning

25.
Explain why *-itis* in tendonitis is called a suffix.

_____

_____.

OK, let's review what you've covered.

26.

root

The fundamental base from which meaningful terms grow or are formed is called the _____.

27.

prefix

A meaningful word or unit placed in front of a root or word is a

_____.

28.

suffix

A syllable or word part joined to the end of a root or word and changes its meaning is a _____.

29.

combining form

When a vowel (a, e, i, o, u) is added to a word root, the word part resulting is called the _____ _____.

30.

compound word

When two or more word roots combine to form a meaningful word, that word is called a _____.

List of Illustrations

(All illustrations created by Sakrantip Blazicek of Ocala, Florida)

1 Basic Word Roots and Common Suffixes

In Unit 1 you will work with basic word roots and a handful of common suffixes. (These are listed in the Mini-Glossary, below.) You'll examine many compound medical terms and discover meanings for all the parts. You'll practice adding various endings to roots and combining forms. By study and practice you'll make more than 30 meaningful medical terms.

Mini-Glossary

acr/o (*extremities*)

cardi/o (*heart*)

cyan/o (*blue*)

cyt/o (*cell*)

dermat/o, derm/o (*skin*)

duoden/o (*duodenum*)

electr/o (*electrical*)

eti/o (*cause*)

gastr/o (*stomach*)

gram/o (*record*)

leuk/o (*white*)

megal/o (*enlarged*)

path/o (*disease*)

-algia (*pain*)

-ectomy (*excision of*)

-itis (*inflammation of*)

-ologist (*one who studies, a specialist*)

-ology (study of)

-osis, -a, -y (condition of, usually abnormal)

-ostomy (forming a new opening)

-otomy (incision into)

-tome (instrument that cuts)

1.
Acr/o means extremities (arms, legs, and the head). To refer to one or more extremities physicians use words containing
_____ / _____.

acr/o

2.
Extremities are the parts of the body farthest from the center of the body. You could say these parts are located on the extreme ends of the main body. What parts are they?

arms, legs, and head

_____.

3.
Extremities in the human body are also known as limbs. When referring to the arms or legs we use the word acr/o. What term could designate the head as an extremity?

acr, acr/o

_____.

4.
When you read a term containing acr or acr/o (the combining form), it should make you think of _____.

extremities or limbs

5.
Each of the terms acr/o/megaly, acr/o/cyan/osis, and acr/o/der-mat/itis has a common word root that refers to what parts of the body? _____, _____, and _____.

arms, legs, head

Write the combining form of the word root meaning extremities.

acr/o

_____

6.
Megal/o means enlarged or oversized. A word containing megal/o means the part or organ of the body is _____

oversized, big, or
   enlarged

_____.

7.
The suffix -*y* denotes a condition, usually abnormal. Acr/o/megal/y means the patient's abnormal condition involves extremities that are

enlargement of,
   oversized, or
   enlarged

_____.

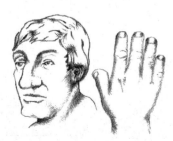

Figure 1.1 Acromegaly

acr/o/megal/y
acromegaly
ak rō meg′ a lē

8.
The illustration on page 2 shows a man with abnormally large hands and head. The term that describes this man's abnormal condition is

_____ / _____ / _____ / _____.

9.
Occasionally you may see a person with very large hands, feet, nose, and chin. The abnormal condition may be

acro/megaly

_____ / _____.

10.
Here are two new suffixes:
-ologist means one who studies, a specialist
-itis means inflammation of (something)
dermat/o refers to the skin.

skin

A dermat/ologist is a specialist in the field of medicine who specializes in treating disease of the _____.

inflammation of the
    skin

Dermat/itis means _____.

Underline the word root in the following medical terms.

Write what each means.

Dermat<u>itis</u>

Dermatitis means _____.

Dermat<u>ologist</u>

Dermatologist means _____.

Now, circle the suffix in each term.

11.
Acrodermatitis is a term meaning inflammation of the skin of the extremities. A person displaying red, inflamed hands may have a condition of

acr/o/dermat/itis
acrodermatitis
ak rō der′ ma tī′ tis

_____ / _____ / _____ / _____.

12.
A busy homemaker may experience an inflammatory condition of her hands and lower arms. The physician may describe this abnormal condition as _____.

acrodermatitis

13.
Remembering that the term acrodermatitis means inflammation of the skin of the extremities, explain the following:

inflammation of
extremities
skin

-itis is a suffix that means _____,

acr/o refers to _____,

dermat is the root for _____.

14.
Cyan/o means blue or blueness. The suffix *-osis* denotes an abnormal condition. Cyan/osis means an abnormal condition of blueness.

abnormal blueness of
the extremities

What do you think acr/o/cyan/osis means? _____
_____.

cyan or cyan/o

The part of the medical term that tells you the color blue is present is _____.

-osis

The part of the medical term denoting that an abnormal condition exists is the suffix _____.

15.

-osis

To denote an abnormal condition, use the suffix _____.

condition
extremities

Acrocyanosis may be defined as the abnormal _____
of blueness of the _____.

16.
Blueness of the extremities is usually due to a reduced amount of oxygen supply to the hands and feet. If the lungs don't take in enough oxygen or the heart doesn't pump enough good blood around the body, the patient's hands and feet may exhibit an abnormal condition described as

acr/o/cyan/osis
acrocyanosis
ak rō sī ə nō′sis

_____ / _____ / _____ / _____.

17.
When the lungs cannot move enough oxygen into the blood because of asthma, blueness of the extremities may result. This is

acrocyanosis

another cause of _____.

the condition of
blueness of the
extremities

18.
Acrocyanosis means _____
_____.

19.
Dermat/osis denotes an abnormal skin condition. The suffix that

-osis

means abnormal condition is _____.

20.

cyan/osis
cyanosis
sī ə nō′sis

Osis is a suffix meaning (usually abnormal) condition. Now, build a term that means an abnormal condition of blueness:
_____ / _____.

dermat/osis
dermatosis
der ma tō′sis

21.
Build a term meaning a skin condition (abnormal, of course):
_____ / _____.

22.
The Greek word *tomos* means a piece cut off. From this word we have many words that refer to cutting: ectomy (cut out), otomy (cut into), -tome (an instrument that cuts). A dermatome is an

skin

instrument that cuts _____.

dermat/ome
dermatome
derm′ə tōm

23.
A dermatome is a surgical instrument. When a physician wants a thin slice of a patient's skin for a skin graft, the doctor asks for a
_____ / _____.

a condition of bluish
  discoloration of the
  skin

24.
Dermat, dermat/o refer to the skin. Cyan/o/derm/a means
_____
_____.

a disease or abnormal
  condition of the skin

Dermat/osis means _____
_____.

cyan/o/derm/a
cyanoderma
sī ə nō der′mä

25.
Cyanoderma sometimes occurs when children swim too long in cold water. If a patient has a bluish discoloration of the skin, for any reason, the person may exhibit
_____ / _____ / _____ / _____.

leuk or leuk/o

26.
Leuk/o means white or abnormally white. In the term leuk/o/derm/a, the part that means white is _____.

a condition of white
  skin, or abnormally
  white skin

27.
Leukoderma means _____
_____.

leuk/o/derm/a
leukoderma
loo kō der′ mä

28.
Some people have much less color in their skin than is normal. Their skin is white. They may have
_____ / _____ / _____ / _____.

29.
Cyt/o refers to a cell or cells. *-ology* is a suffix that means the study of.

the study of cells

What does cyt/ology mean? _____.

30.
There are several kinds of cells in blood. One kind is the leuk/o/cyte.

white blood cell

A leukocyte is a _____.

31.
There are several different kinds of cells in the bloodstream. When a physician wants to know how many "infection-fighting" white blood cells are circulating, the doctor asks the lab technician to count the _____ / _____ /cytes.

leuk/o/cyt/e
leukocyte
lōō′ kō sīt

32.
Emia is a suffix meaning blood. When a person's blood contains far too many white blood cells, it may indicate a condition sometimes described as "blood cancer." A term meaning literally *white blood* is _____ / _____.

leuk/emia
leukemia
lōō kē′ mē ə

33.
In the term *acromegaly,* the combining form used for extremities is _____, the word root for oversized is _____, and the suffix meaning *condition of* is _____.

acr/o
megal
y

34.
Now try this. *Cardi/o* means heart. Another suffix meaning condition of is *-a*. What does megal/o/cardi/a mean? _____ _____.

a condition of oversized
   heart, or enlargement
   of the heart

35.
When any muscle exercises, it gets larger. If the heart muscle overexercises, an enlarged condition of the heart may occur. It is described as _____ / _____ / _____ / _____.

megal/o/card/ia
megalocardia
meg ə lō kär′ dē ä

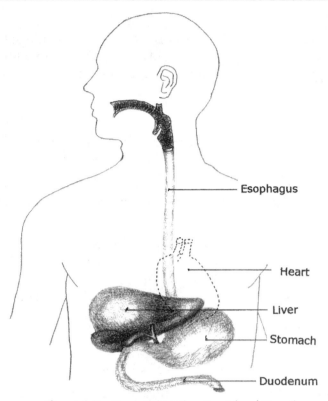

Figure 1.2 Upper Digestive Tract (and Heart)

The Digestive Tract begins with the oral cavity. The teeth pulverize ingested food and soften it. The action of the tongue moves the partly digested food into the *esophagus* by swallowing. Then strong muscular contractions move the food to the *stomach*. In the stomach the food is further processed mechanically and chemically. Then it passes into the highly coiled intestine. The first part of the intestine is called the *duodenum*.

Esophagus (esophag/o)   Stomach (gastr/o)
Duodenum (duoden/o)   Heart (cardi/o)

36.
When the heart muscle doesn't receive an adequate supply of oxygen, the heart may beat more often. Inadequate oxygen makes the heart work harder and may lead to an enlarged heart described as

megalocardia or
cardiomegaly

megal/o/gastr/ia
megalogastria
meg ə lō gas′ trē ä
    OR
gastromegaly
gas′ trō meg′ a lē

37.
Try this one. *Gastr* is the word root for stomach. When the stomach enlarges so that it crowds other organs, an undesirable condition exists known as

_____ / _____ / _____ /ia.
     enlarged   stomach

OR

_____ / _____ / _____ /y.
     stomach   enlarged

oversized heart, or
   enlargement of the
   heart

(the same thing)

38.
Megalocardia means _____
_____.

What does cardiomegaly mean? _____

39.
The suffix *-itis* means inflammation of (something).

inflammation of the
   heart

What does carditis mean? _____
_____

stomach

Both gastr–, gastr/o mean _____.

inflammation of the
   stomach

Gastritis means _____
_____.

40.
Here's a quick review. Using the suggested answers, write the meaning of each of the following terms.

SUGGESTED ANSWERS:

abnormal condition of blueness	heart
cell	inflammation of
cutting instrument	skin
enlarged, oversized	stomach
extremities	white

extremities
blueness
white
stomach
cell
heart

acr/o _____
cyan/o _____
leuk/o _____
gastr/o _____
cyt/o _____
cardi/o _____

enlarged, oversized	megal/o _____
skin	derm/o, dermat/o _____
abnormal condition of	–osis (-a, -y) _____
inflammation of	–itis _____
cutting instrument	–tome _____

41.
Now build a medical term for each of the following:

a condition of oversized extremities

acro/megal/y

_____ / _____ / _____
extremities   oversized

leuko/cyte

a white cell _____ / _____

dermat/itis

inflammation of the skin _____ / _____

megalo/cardi/a
OR
cardio/megal/y

a condition of enlarged heart

_____ / _____ / _____

42.
Let's have a change of pace here. Professional health workers use some special words to talk about illness and sick people. Here are just a few you'll find very useful. Read each definition. Then underline a key word or words to help you remember the meaning of the term.

It's up to you, of course, but here are some key words.

sickness, illness

Disease is a condition in which bodily health is impaired. It means sickness or illness.

exhibition, display, evidence

Manifestation is proof of impaired bodily health. It's a display, exhibition, or evidence of disease.

changes (structural and functional)

Pathology is the scientific study of changes in the human body (structural and functional) produced by disease.

causes (ētēology)

Etiology is the scientific study of causes of disease.

You may refer to the definitions if you need help answering the next few frames.

The cause of the patient's disease is not yet known (and may remain unknown).

43.
If a physician says that a patient's disease is of unknown etiology, what would that mean to you? _____

_____

_____.

sickness, illness

44.
Another word for disease is _____.

evidence, or exhibition

45.
Manifestation is a display, or _____,
of disease.

causes

46.
Etiology is the scientific study of _____ of disease.

structural
functional
disease

47.
Pathology is the scientific study of _____ and
_____ changes in the body produced by
_____.

48.
Select the best term for each definition. Write your choice in the
space provided.

pathology   etiology   manifestation   disease

disease

Another term for illness or sickness is _____.

manifestation

Evidence, or proof, of disease is _____.

etiology

The study of causes of disease is _____.

pathology

The scientific study of changes in the body produced by disease is
_____.

path/ologist
pathologist
path ol′ ə jist

49.
The suffix -*ology* means the study of, the suffix -*ologist* means one
who studies (and becomes an expert). One who studies structural
and functional changes in the body produced by disease is a
_____ / _____.

cardi/ologist
cardiologist
kär dē ol′ ə jist

50.
Some physicians specialize in heart disease. The specialist
who determines that a heart is deformed is a
_____ / _____.
            heart   specialist

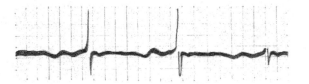

Figure 1.3   Electrocardiography (ECG)

Electrocardiography is a method of recording electrical currents traversing the heart muscle just prior to each heart beat. An Electrocardiogram is a graphic record of heart action currents that are obtained by electrocardiography.

cardiologist

51.
A heart doctor who reads an electr/o/cardi/o/gram (a record of electrical impulses generated by the heart) is a specialist in heart problems or _____ / _____.

a record of electrical
    waves given off by
    the heart (or
    equivalent)

52.
Complete the meaning of electr/o/cardi/o/gram:

Gram means a record or recording, electr/o means _____

_____

_____

heart

cardi/o means _____

electr/o/cardi/o/gram
electrocardiogram
ē lek′ trō kär′ dē ə
    gram

53.
The electr/o/cardi/o/gram is a record obtained by electr/o/cardi/o/graph/y. A technician can learn electrocardiography, but it takes a cardiologist to read the
_____ / _____ / _____ / _____ / _____.
    electrical   heart   record

54.

A physician specialist can look at a report that looks like this

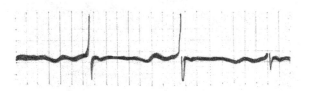

Figure 1.4   Electrocardiogram (ECG)

and learn something about a patient's heart function. This specialist
is probably a _____ and can read an

cardiologist
electrocardiogram

_____.
         (ECG)

cardi/algia
cardialgia
kär dē al′ jē a (There is
   no need to add a
   vowel to the root
   cardi because –algia
   begins with a vowel.)

55.

The suffix *-algia* means pain. Form a word that means heart pain:

_____ / _____.
         heart   pain

cardialgia

56.

When a patient complains of pain in the heart, the symptom is
known medically as _____.

57.

Gastralgia means pain in the stomach.

stomach

Gastr is the root for _____.

–algia

The suffix for pain is _____.

58.

Gastr/ectomy means excision (removal) of all or part of the stomach. Gastr means _____.

stomach

to cut out, excise, or
   remove surgically

The suffix *-ectomy* means _____

_____.

59.

gastr/ectomy
gastrectomy
gas trek′ tō mē

When a patient's stomach ulcer perforates, the surgeon may need to remove part of the stomach. The medical term for the procedure is

_____ / _____.
(stomach)   (excision of)

60.

gastrectomy

Cancer of the stomach may require a surgeon to remove all or part of the patient's stomach. This procedure is a _____.

61.

gastr/itis
gastritis
gas trī′ tis

Form a word that means inflammation of the stomach.

_____ / _____.

62.

duoden/um
duodenum
dōo ōd′ nəm (or
  dōo ō dē′ nəm)

The stomach emptics its contents into the first section of the intestine, called the duodenum. *Duoden* is the word root for

_____.

gastr

What is the root for stomach? _____.

63.

stomach and
  duodenum

The suffix -*ostomy* means a procedure to form a new opening. Gastr/o/duoden/ostomy means forming a new opening between the _____ and _____.

64.

gastr/o/duoden/
  ostomy
gastroduodenostomy
gas′ trō dōo ō de nos′
  tō mē

A surgeon may need to remove a portion of a diseased stomach. If the natural connection is removed, then the surgeon must form a new opening between the stomach and duodenum. This procedure is called

_____ / _____ / _____ / _____.

65.

a surgical procedure to
  form a new opening
  between the stomach
  and duodenum

When an abnormal condition exists between the stomach and the duodenum, a surgeon may need to perform a gastroduodenostomy, which means _____
_____
_____

duodenum
dū ō dē′ num

66.
The suffix -ectomy means excision of; -ostomy means forming a new opening. The form *-otomy* means incision into. A duo/den/otomy is an incision into the _____.

-otomy

duoden/otomy
duodenotomy
dōō od ə not′ ə mē

67.
The suffix for incision into is _____.

If a physician makes an incision into the wall of the duodenum, the doctor has performed a _____ / _____.

-itis

duoden/itis
duodenitis
dōō od ə nī′ tis

68.
The suffix for inflammation is _____.

The word for inflammation of the duodenum is _____ / _____.

69.
Duoden/al means of or pertaining to the duodenum.

-al is a suffix meaning of, or pertaining to. Therefore matern/al

of, or pertaining to,
    mother; of, or
    pertaining to, father

means _____ and patern/al means _____ _____.

duoden/al
duodenal
dōō ō dē′ nəl

70.
In the sentence "Duodenal carcinoma was present," the word meaning of, or pertaining to, the duodenum is _____ / _____.

duoden/ostomy
duodenostomy
dōō od ə nos′ tō mē

71.
The suffix -ostomy means making a new opening. The word to form a new opening into the duodenum is _____ / _____.

gastroduodenostomy

72.
Here's one for you to figure out. A duodenostomy can be formed in more than one manner. If it is formed with the stomach, it is called a _____.

stomach	duodenum	new opening

-ostomy

73.
The suffix for forming a new opening is _____.

74.
Let's review what you've covered. Using the suggested answers, write the meaning of each of the following terms.

SUGGESTED ANSWERS:

blueness	duodenum
cell	electrical
cause(s)	enlarged, oversized
changes due to disease	record of

duodenum   duoden/o _____

changes due to disease   path/o _____.

record of   gram/o _____

cell   cyt/o _____

electric   electr/o _____

cause   eti/o _____

enlarged, oversized   megal/o _____

blueness   cyan/o _____

75.
Now try it with the suffixes you just learned.

SUGGESTED ANSWERS:

(abnormal) condition of	incision into
cutting instrument	inflammation of
form a new opening	of, or pertaining to
one who studies, specializes in	pain

of, or pertaining to   –al _____

inflammation of   –itis _____

(abnormal) condition   –osis, –a, –y _____

form a new opening   –ostomy _____

cutting instrument   –tome _____

incision into   –otomy _____

pain   –algia _____

one who studies   –ologist _____

cyan/osis

76.
Now build some new words.
A condition of blueness is _____ / _____.
　　　　　　　　　　　　　　　blueness　　　　　　　　　　condition

path/ologist

One who studies bodily changes produced by disease is a
_____ / _____.
changes in the body　　　　　　one who studies

duoden/ostomy

A surgical procedure that forms a new opening in the duodenum is
a _____ / _____.
　　　　　duodenum　　　　　　form a new opening

eti/o/logic/al

A term meaning of, or pertaining to, the study of causes of disease
is _____ / _____ / _____ / _____.
causes of disease　　　　　　　　the study of　　　　pertaining to

77.
While working through Unit 1, you formed the following new
medical terms. Read them one at a time and pronounce each aloud
several times until you can articulate each term clearly and correctly.
If a friend pronounces each term for you, could you spell it correctly? Try it.

acrocyanosis (ak rō sī ə nō′ sis)　　dermatologist
acrodermatitis　　　　　　　　　　　(der ma tol′ ə jist)
　　(ak rō der′ ma tī′tis)　　　　　dermatome (derm′ ə tōm)
acromegaly (ak rō meg′ a lē)　　　dermatosis (der ma tō′ sis)
cardialgia (kär dē al′ jē a)　　　disease (diz ēz′)
cardiologist (kär dē ol′ ə jist)　duodenal (do͞o ō dē′ nəl)
carditis (kär dī′ tis)　　　　　　electrocardiogram
cyanoderma (sī ə nō der′ mä)　　　(ē lek′ trō kär′ dē ə gram)
cyanosis (sī ə nō′ sis)　　　　　　etiological (ē′ tē ō loj′ i kəl)
cytology (sī tol′ ə jē)　　　　　gastralgia (gas tral′ jē a)
gastrectomy　　　　　　　　　　　manifestation
　　(gas trek′ tō mē)　　　　　　　(man′ ə fes tā′ shən)
gastritis (gas trī′ tis)　　　　megalocardia
gastroduodenostomy　　　　　　　(meg ə lō kär′ dē ä)
　　(gas′ trō do͞o ō de nos′ tō mē)　megalogastria
leukemia (lo͞o kē′ mē ə)　　　　　(meg ə lō gas′ trē ä)
leukocyte (lo͞o′ kō sīt)　　　　pathologist (path ol′ ə jist)
leukoderma (lo͞o kō der′ mä)　　pathology (path ol′ ə jē)

Before going on to Unit 2, take the Unit 1 Self-Test that follows.

Unit 1 Self-Test

Part 1

From the list of definitions on the right, select the correct meaning for each of the terms in the left-hand column. Write the letter in the space provided.

_____ 1. Megalocardia

_____ 2. Cardiology

_____ 3. Duodenostomy

_____ 4. Leukemia

_____ 5. Dermatologist

_____ 6. Electrocardiography

_____ 7. Acromegaly

_____ 8. Gastritis

_____ 9. Dermatome

_____ 10. Manifestation

_____ 11. Gastroduodenostomy

_____ 12. Etiology

_____ 13. Acrocyanosis

_____ 14. Pathologist

_____ 15. Gastralgia

a. Study of, or pertaining to, causes (of disease)

b. A specialist in the field of skin diseases

c. A condition of blueness of the extremities

d. Enlargement of the heart

e. A surgical procedure forming a new opening in the duodenum

f. Display, evidence of disease

g. One who specializes in the study of structural and functional changes in the body

h. Pain in the stomach

i. Inflammation of the stomach

j. Recordings of electrical waves of the heart

k. An abnormal condition of enlarged extremities

l. A surgical instrument for cutting skin

m. A surgical operation to make a new opening between the stomach and duodenum

n. The study of disease of the heart

o. An abnormal condition of too many white blood cells

Part 2

Write a medical term for each of the following:

1. Impaired bodily health   _____

2. Bluish discoloration of the skin   _____

3. White cell   _____

4. Oversized or enlarged stomach   _____

5. Evidence of disease   _____

6. The study of causes of an illness   _____

7. Excision or removal of the stomach   _____

8. Pertaining to the duodenum   _____

9. Generalized condition of blueness   _____

10. Heart pain   _____

11. Inflammation of the heart   _____

12. An abnormal condition of white skin   _____

13. Inflammation of the skin of the extremities   _____

14. Study of cell(s)   _____

15. An abnormal condition of the skin   _____

ANSWERS

Part 1	Part 2
1. d	1. disease
2. n	2. cyanoderma
3. e	3. leukocyte
4. o	4. megalogastria
5. b	5. manifestation
6. j	6. etiology
7. k	7. gastrectomy
8. i	8. duodenal
9. l	9. cyanosis
10. f	10. cardialgia

11. m	11. carditis
12. a	12. leukoderma
13. c	13. acrodermatitis
14. g	14. cytology
15. h	15. dermatosis

2 More Word Roots, Suffixes, and Prefixes

In Unit 2 you will cover more sophisticated terms, word roots, and suffixes, and you'll begin using prefixes. Teaching sequences in this unit aim to expand your learning by combining words you covered in Unit 1 with some new ones. We introduced new ideas as well as useful medical terms to improve retention and make your practice exercises interesting. Now, let's get started.

Mini-Glossary

aden/o (*gland*)

arthr/o (*joint*)

carcin/o (*malignancy*)

cele/o, o/cele (*hernia*)

cephal/o (*head*)

chondr/o (*cartilage*)

cost/o (*ribs*)

dent/o (*tooth*)

emes/is (*vomiting*)

hist/o (*tissue*)

laryng/o (*larynx*)

lip/o (*fat*)

malac/o (*soft*)

morph/o (*structure* of)

muc/o (*mucus*)

onc/o (*tumor*)

ost/o, oste/o (*bone*)

plast/o (*repair*)

trach/e (*trachea*)

troph/o (*development*)

en-, endo- (*in, inside, within*)

ex-, ex/o- (*outside, out*)

hyper- (*excessive*)

hypo- (*under*)

inter- (*between*)

-al, -ar, -ic (*of, or pertaining to*)

-oid (*resembling*)

-oma (*tumor*)

-ism (medical condition, disease)

Before you begin Unit 2, complete the Review Sheet for Unit 1. It will help you get a running start as you continue your studying. You'll find review sheets beginning on page 247.

1.
Examine the terms hyper/trophy, hyper/emia, and hyper/emesis. *Hyper-* means excessive, more than normal amount. Hyper- placed in front of trophy, emia, and emesis changes the meaning of the terms. Therefore, hyper- is a _____ (prefix/suffix?).

prefix

2.
Hyper/thyroid/ism is a medical condition of the thyroid gland resulting in excessive thyroid gland activity. The prefix expressing higher than normal activity of the thyroid gland is _____.

hyper

3.
The suffix *-ism* indicates there is a medical condition involving some specified thing or body part. In the case of hyper/thyroid/ism the medical condition involves what body part? _____.

thyroid gland

Here's a suggestion: Hyperthyroidism means the patient has a medical condition resulting from excessive activity of the thyroid gland.

4.
Hyper- means something is excessive. Thyroid tells you what part is involved. The suffix -ism means there is a resulting medical condition.

In your words, explain the meaning of the term hyper/thyroid/ism.

_____
_____
_____.

5.
Emesis is a word that means vomiting. A word that means excessive vomiting is _____ / _____.

hyper/emesis
hyperemesis
hī per em′ ə sis

Gallbladder attacks can cause excessive vomiting. This, too, is called

hyperemesis

_____.

6.
Hyper/trophy means overdevelopment; *troph/o* comes from the Greek word for nourishment. Note the connection between nourishment and development. Overdevelopment is called

hyper/troph/y
hypertrophy
hī per′ trō fē

_____ / _____ /y.
a condition of excessive development

hypertrophy

Muscles also can overdevelop or _____.
(a verb form)

hypertrophy

7.
Many organs can overdevelop. If the heart overdevelops, the condition is called cardiac _____.

hypo-

8.
The prefix *hypo-* is just the opposite of hyper-. The prefix for under or less than normal is _____.

skin

skin

9.
Derm/o refers to the _____. The suffix -ic means of, or pertaining to. Hypo/derm/ic means pertaining to under the

_____.

hypo/derm/ic
hypodermic
hī pō der′ mik

10.
A hypodermic needle is short because it goes just under the skin. A shot given superficially is administered with a

_____ / _____ / _____ needle.
     under   skin   pertaining to

aden/itis
adenitis
ad ə nī′ tis

11.
Aden/o is used in words that refer to glands. Build a word that means inflammation of a gland:
_____ / _____.
    gland   inflammation of

aden/ectomy
adenectomy
ad ə nek′ tō mē

12.
Since ectomy means excision (or surgical removal of), the word for surgical removal of a gland is
_____ / _____.
    gland   surgical removal

adenectomy

13.
If a gland is like a tumor, part or all of it may be excised. Excision of a gland is _____.

aden/oma
adenoma
ad ə nō′ mä

14.
The suffix *-oma* means tumor. Form a word that means tumor of a gland:
_____ / _____.

surgical removal, or
excision, of the
thyroid gland

15.
Try this. Sometimes the thyroid gland develops a tumor. A patient's history might read, ". . . because of the presence of a thyroid adenoma, thyroidectomy is indicated." What is a thyroid/ectomy?

_____

_____.

16.
The suffixes *-ic, -al,* and *-ar* mean of, or pertaining to, the attached word.

spleen

A splenic tumor is a tumor of the _____.

tonsil

A tonsillar tumor is a tumor pertaining to the _____.

Where would you expect to find a duodenal tumor? _____

in the duodenum

_____.

17.
Carcin/o is the root for cancer. The suffix –oma means tumor. A

cancerous tumor

carcinoma is a _____.

18.
A carcinoma may occur in almost any part of the body. A cancerous

splenic

tumor of the spleen is called _____ carcinoma.

carcinoma

Cancer of the tonsil is tonsillar _____.

of, or pertaining to

The suffixes –ic, –ar, and –al mean _____.

19.

tumor

An adenoma is a glandular tumor; –oma means _____.

A lip/oma is a tumor of fatty tissue.

fat, fatty tissue

Lip/o is the combining form for _____.

lip/oma
lipoma
li po' ma

20.
A fatty tumor is called a _____ / _____.

lip/oid
lipoid
lip' oid

21.
Lipoma is a fatty tumor; *-oid* is a suffix meaning like or resembling. Using the word root for fatty tissue, build a term that means fatlike, or resembling fat: _____ / _____.

22.
The word lipoid is used in chemistry and pathology. It describes a substance that looks like fat, dissolves like fat, but is not fat. Cholesterol is an alcohol that resembles fat; therefore, cholesterol is a

lip/oid

_____ / _____ substance.
       fat   like

muc/oid
mucoid
my$\overline{oo}$′ koid

23.
Muc/oid means resembling mucus. There is a substance in connective tissue that resembles mucus. This is called a
_____ / _____ substance.

24.
There is a protein in the body that is said to be mucoid in nature.

resembling mucus

Mucoid means _____.

25.
A substance that resembles mucus is best described as

mucoid

_____.

lipoid

A substance resembling fatty tissue is called a _____ substance.

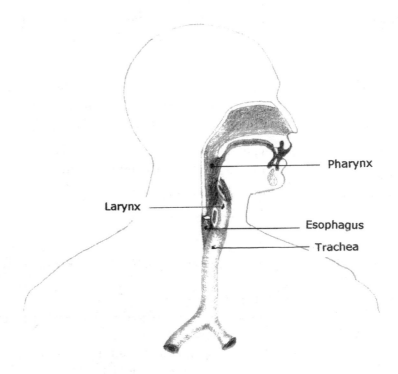

Figure 2.1 The Upper Respiratory Tract

The Respiratory Tract conducts oxygen-rich air to the lungs where oxygen can be readily absorbed by the blood. It removes carbon dioxide–laden air to the external atmosphere. The *pharynx* filters and warms the air we breathe and conducts it into the *larynx*. The larynx protects against inadvertent inhaling of solid matter and contains the vocal cords, the mechanism of sound production. Leading from the larynx is the windpipe, more correctly known as the *trachea*.

Pharynx (pharyng/o)   Trachea (trache/o)
Larynx (laryng/o)

26.
The larynx or *voice box* contains the vocal cords. *Laryng/o* is the combining form for building words referring to the voice box, also called the _____.

larynx

laryng/itis
laryngitis
lair an jī′ tis

Build a term meaning inflammation of the larynx.
_____ / _____.

inflammation of the
  larynx

27.
After a bad cold, a patient may develop laryngitis, which means
_____.

28.
Now, you'll add a few new suffixes to your growing vocabulary. An obstruction of the colon may require a new opening into the colon that will be *permanent*.

(kō los′ tō mē)

a new (permanent)
  opening into the
  colon

Col, col/o refer to the colon, or large bowel. The suffix *-ostomy* means a new (permanent) opening into.

Col/ostomy means _____
_____.

29.
The suffix for a new (permanent) opening is _____.

-ostomy

30.
Take a look at Illustration 2.1. An obstruction of the windpipe makes breathing very difficult, or even impossible. In an emergency, a physician may make an incision into the windpipe to permit a free flow of air to the patient's lungs.

(trā kē ot′ ō mē)

an incision into, or
  temporary opening
  into, the trachea, or
  windpipe

Trache, trache/o refer to the trachea, or *windpipe*. The suffix -otomy means incision into, or a *temporary* opening.

Trache/otomy means _____
_____.

-otomy

31.
The suffix meaning a temporary opening, or incision into, is

_____.

-ostomy

32.
Which suffix would you use to indicate creation of a new (permanent) opening? _____.

-otomy

Which suffix means making an incision into, or creating a temporary opening? _____.

creation of a new
   (permanent) opening
   into the colon

33.
Colostomy means _____

_____.

incision into, or
   temporary opening
   into, the trachea

Tracheotomy means _____

_____.

34.
Time for a quick review. Using the suggested answers, write a meaning for each of the following word roots.

SUGGESTED ANSWERS:

fat, fatty	mucus
larynx	skin
cancer, malignant	spleen

fat, fatty
spleen
skin
larynx
mucus
cancer, malignant

lip/o _____

splen/o _____

derm/o _____

laryng/o _____

muc/o _____

carcin/o _____

35.
Now do the same with the following suffixes.

SUGGESTED ANSWERS:

incision into, temporary opening	a new (permanent) opening into
like, or resembling	development
of or pertaining to	vomiting
tumor	excision of

development
excision of

-trophy _____.

-ectomy _____.

incision into,
    temporary opening   –otomy _____

a new (permanent)
    opening into   –ostomy _____

of, or pertaining to   –ic, –ar, –al _____

like, or resembling   –oid _____

vomiting   –emesis _____

tumor   –oma _____

36.
Complete the following:

under, less   Hypo- is a prefix meaning _____.

over, excessive   Hyper- is a prefix meaning _____.

37.
Build a medical term for each of the following:

muc/oid   resembling mucus _____ / _____.
                            mucus   like

splen/ic   pertaining to the spleen _____ / _____.
                             spleen   of the

aden/ectomy   excision of a gland _____ / _____.
                           gland   excision of

hyper/trophy   overdevelopment _____ / _____.
                             excessive   development

hypo/derm/ic   under the skin _____ / _____ / _____..
                           under   skin   pertaining to

                new (permanent) opening into the larynx

laryng/ostomy   _____ / _____.
                      larynx   new opening

38.
Here are two terms to define.

a condition of excess
    development,
    oversized   Hypertrophy means _____

                _____.

of, or pertaining to,
    under the skin   Hypodermal means _____

                _____.

This is a good place to stop and take a short break.

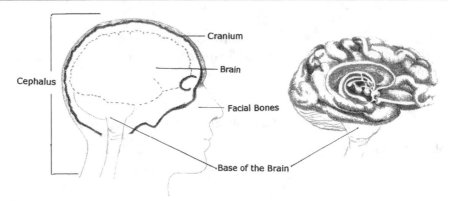

Figure 2.2   The Head

Cephalus is a term that refers to the entire head. It is composed of both the cranium and facial bones. The *cranium* (or skull) is a bony vault protecting the contents of the head. The face is the front portion of the head and includes the eyes, nose, mouth, forehead, cheeks, and chin. The cranium encloses the *cerebrum,* also known as the brain. The brain is the center of sensory awareness and movement, emotions, rational thought and behavior, foresight and planning, memory, speech, language, and interpretation of language.

Cephalus, head including skull and facial bones (cephal/o)
Cranium (crani/o)
Cerebrum (cerebr/o)

Use the illustration of the head to help you with the frames that follow.

39.
Welcome back. At this stage of word-building, students sometimes find they have one big headache. Both ceph/algia and cephal/algia mean pain in the head. The combining form and root for head are

cephal/o
ceph

_____ and _____.

40.
To indicate pain we use –algia. Any headache may be called

ceph/algia or
cephal/algia
cephalalgia
(sef ə lal′ jē ä)

_____ / _____ or
      head   pain

_____ / _____.
      head   ache

41.
The word root and combining form for head is *ceph, cephal/o*. Two words for pain in the head are _____

cephalalgia
  and cephalgia

_____.

42.
headache

Cephalalgia means _____.

of, or pertaining to, the
  head

Cephal/ic means _____

_____.

cephal/ic
cephalic
sə fal' ik

43.
A case history reporting head wounds due to an accident might read, "_____ / _____ lacerations were present."

cephalic

44.
A tumor located on the head might be noted as a _____ tumor.

Prefix	Meaning
en-, endo-	in, inside, within
ex-, exo-	out, outside completely

Use the table to help with the frames that follow.

inside the head (the
  brain)

45.
Cephal/o means head. What does *en*cephal/o mean?

_____.

brain

46.
Since the brain is enclosed inside the head's bony vault, encephal/o means the organ inside the head, or the _____.

47.
Using the word root for head, build words meaning the following:
inflammation of the brain

encephal/itis
en sef ə lī' tis

_____ / _____.
      brain   inflammation of

encephal/oma
en sef' ə lō' mä

brain tumor _____ / _____.
        brain   tumor of

inflammation within
  the heart

48.
What does endocarditis mean? _____

_____.

ex-, exo-

49.
Refer to Frame 44 for help. Select a prefix meaning out, or completely outside of: _____.
en-, endo- or ex-, exo-

50.
Exo/genous means originating completely outside of an organ or part. *Genous* takes its meaning from a Latin word meaning to produce or originate.

exo-

What part of the term means completely outside of? _____.

exo/genous
ex′ oj′ ə nus

Something originating completely outside of an organism, cell, or organ is called _____ / _____.
outside   produced or originating

endo/genous
en′ doj′ ə nus

Now build a word that indicates something is produced or originates from within a cell or organism:
_____ / _____.
within   produced or originating

51.
Try these. Here are some common English words often used in the medical world. Write what each means.

hale (breathe)   cise (cut)   spire (breathe)

breathe out

exhale means _____.

cut out

excise means _____ _____.

breathe out (it also
  means to die or
  breathe out for the
  last time)

expire means _____.

52.
Write two forms of a prefix for each of the following.

en-, endo-

in, inside of, within _____, _____.

ex-, exo-

out, completely outside of _____, _____.

53.
The Greek word for hernia is *kele*. From this we derive the combining forms *cele/o* or *o/cele*. Encephal/o/cele is a word meaning

brain

herniation of _____ tissue.

encephal/o/cele
encephalocele
en səf′ a lō sēl

54.
Any hernia is a protrusion of a part from its natural cavity.
Herniation is expressed by cele. A protrusion of brain tissue
from its natural cavity is an

_____ / _____ / _____.
     brain (inside the head)   hernia

encephalocele

55.
Increased fluid inside the head sometimes causes herniation at the
base of the brain. Herniation of the brain in medical language is
called an _____.

a condition of softened
brain tissue

56.
Malac/ia is a word meaning soft, or softened, tissue.
Encephal/o/malac/ia means _____

_____.

encephal/o/malac/ia
encephalomalacia
en sef′ a lō mä la′ zhə

57.
Malac/o is the combining form for soft, or softened. The term
meaning softened brain tissue is

_____ / ____ / _____ / ___ia___.
      brain tissue   softened   a condition of

encephalomalacia

58.
An accident causing brain injury could result in softened brain
tissue, called _____.

oste/itis
osteitis
os tē ī′ tis

59.
Oste is the root referring to bone. A word meaning inflammation of
the bone is _____ / _____.

a condition of softened
bone tissue

60.
What do you think oste/o/malac/ia means? _____

_____.

oste/o/malac/ia
osteomalacia
os′ tē ō mä lā′ zhə

61.
Insufficient calcium in a young person's diet may lead to gradual
softening and bending of bones. This disorder is called

_____ / _____ / _____ / _____.
     bone   softened   condition

62.
A disorder of the parathyroid gland can cause calcium to be withdrawn from bones. The resulting condition may be called

osteomalacia

_____.

63.

oste/oma
osteoma
os tē ō′ mä

A hard outgrowth on any bone could be a bone tumor. In medical terms, it would be referred to as an

_____ / _____.

a tumor inside (the center canal of the bone)

What does end/oste/oma mean? _____

_____.

64.
Arthr/o refers to joints; _plast/y_ means surgical repair of. What does

surgical repair of a joint(s)

arthr/o/plast/y mean? _____

_____.

65.
Think of a plastic surgeon building a new nose or doing a face lift. These are surgical repairs or restoration. When a joint has lost its ability to move, movement can sometimes be restored by an

arthr/o/plast/y
arthroplasty
arth′ rō plas′ tē

_____ / ___ / _____ / __y_____.
       joint   repair or restore   (process/procedure)

66.

arthro/plasty

If a child is born without a joint, sometimes one can be formed by a surgical procedure called _____ / _____.

arthr/itis
arthritis
ärth rī′ tis

67.
Form a word that means inflammation of a joint:

_____ / _____.
      joint   inflammation of

arthr/otomy
arthrotomy
ärth rot′ ō mē

68.
Now form a word that means incision into a joint:

_____ / _____.
      joint   temporary opening

69.
The word oste/o/chondr/itis means inflammation of the bone and cartilage. The word root for cartilage must be

chondr   _____.

bone   Oste, oste/o mean _____.

70.
Analyze oste/o/chondr/itis:

oste/o   combining form for bone is _____

chondr   word root for cartilage is _____

–itis   suffix for inflammation is _____

oste/o/chondr/itis
osteochondritis
os′ tē ō kon drī′ tis

71.
Now put all the parts together:
_____ / _____ / _____ / _____.
            bone   cartilage   inflammation of

inflammation of bone
    and cartilage

What does osteochondritis mean? _____
_____.

excision of cartilage

72.
Chondr/ectomy means _____
_____.

inter-
of or pertaining to

73.
Cost/al means pertaining to the ribs. *Inter/cost/al* means pertaining to between the ribs. The prefix for between is _____.
The suffix –al means _____.

inter/cost/al
intercostal
in ter kos′ t′l

74.
There are short strong muscles between the ribs. These muscles move the ribs during breathing and are called
_____ / _____ / _____ muscles.
           between   ribs

intercostal

75.
One set of between-the-ribs muscles enlarges the rib cage when breathing in. When exhaling, the rib cage is made smaller by another set of _____ muscles.
                 (between-the-ribs)

teeth
teeth

spaces between the
   teeth

76.
A *dent*/ist takes care of _____. A dent/ifrice is used
for cleaning _____.

Interdental spaces means _____
_____.

dent/algia
dentalgia
den tal′ jē a

dent/oid
dentoid
den′ toid

77.
Try making a few new words. Pain in the teeth, or a toothache, is
called _____ / _____.

A word that means tooth-shaped or resembling a tooth is
_____ / _____.

(If you're not sure, use
   your dictionary.)

78.
Try these. Pathogenic means something that produces disease.

What is a pathogenic organism? _____

What does pathology mean? _____

Therefore, pathological means _____
_____.

Excessive vomiting is
   evidence of a
   diseased condition.

A graphic representation
   of brain activity
   (EEG) is necessary to
   determine the cause
   of brain disease (or
   something similar in
   your words).

79.
Explain each of the following statements in simple language.

Hyperemesis is a manifestation of a pathological condition. _____
_____

Electroencephalography (EEG) is often the first step toward a diagnosis of encephalopathy. _____
_____
_____
_____

80.

It's time to review again. Using the suggested answers, write the meaning of each of the following terms.

SUGGESTED ANSWERS:

bone	joint
cartilage	rib
head	soft, soften
hernia	tooth, teeth

joint	arthr/o _____.
hernia	cele/o _____.
head	cephal/o _____.
cartilage	chondr/o _____.
rib	cost/o _____.
tooth, teeth	dent/o _____.
soft, soften	malac/o _____.
bone	ost-, oste-, oste/o _____.

81.

These word parts are used as suffixes.

repair of (restoration or plastic surgery)	–plasty means _____.
hernia (protrusion of a part from its natural cavity)	–cele means _____ _____.

82.

Here are some easy ones.

in, within, inside	end–, endo– is a prefix meaning _____.
out, completely outside of	ex–, exo– is a prefix meaning _____.

83.

Build a medical term for each of the following.

arthro/plasty	restoration of a joint _____ / _____. joint plastic surgery of
inter/costal	between the ribs _____ / _____. between ribs
chondro/malacia	softening of cartilage _____ / _____. cartilage softened
oste/oma	bony tumor _____ / _____. bone tumor of

encephalo/cele   herniation of the brain _____ / _____.
                                                 inside the head   hernia of

dent/oid   resembling teeth _____ / _____.
                                               teeth   resembling

ceph/algia   headache _____ / _____.
                                       head   pain

arthr/otomy   incision into a joint _____ / _____.
                                                    joint   temporary opening

84.

You just learned the suffix –oma, meaning tumor. Now, here are three more very useful terms often used in discussion of tumors.

Here are our suggestions:

Read each definition. Then underline a key word or two to help you remember what the term means.

tumors, branch of medicine

Oncology is the branch of medicine dealing with tumors.

structure of an organ, part

Morphology is the biological science dealing with the structure of an organ or part of the body.

microscopic tissues of a part

Histology is the study of the microscopic tissues that make up a part or a structure.

changes caused by disease

Pathology is the study of changes in structure and function caused by disease.

85.

Complete each of the following statements. Look back at the definition if necessary.

tumors   Onc/o refers to _____.

tissues (of a part, organ)   Hist/o refers to _____.

changes (due to disease)   Path/o refers to _____.

structure (of an organ, part) Morph/o refers to _____.

86.

Complete each definition.

structure   Morphology is the study of the _____ of an organ or part.

tissues   Histology is the study of microscopic _____ making up a part or structure.

tumors   Oncology is the study of _____.

changes   Pathology is the study of _____ caused by disease.

87.

Complete each of the following definitions:

One who studies the tissue *structure* under a microscope is a

histologist _____.

A specialist in the care and treatment of patients with *tumors* is an

oncologist _____.

One who studies the *structure* of living organisms is a

morphologist _____.

A specialist who studies *changes* in structure and function resulting

pathologist from disease is a _____.

88.

Here are more than 30 medical terms you worked with in Unit 2.
Read each one. Say it aloud several times and explain what it means
aloud (so your ears and brain can hear what you learned).

adenectomy (ad ə nek′ tō mē)
adenitis (ad ə nī′ tis)
adenoma (ad ə nō′ mä)
arthroplasty (ärth′ rō plas′ tē)
arthrotomy (ärth rot′ ō mē)
carcinoma (kär sin ō′ mä)
cephalalgia (sef ə lal′ jē ä)
cephalic (se fal′ ik)
chondritis (kon drī′ tis)
colostomy (kō los′ tō mē)
dentalgia (den tal′ jē ä)
encephalitis (en sef ə lī′ tis)
encephalocele (en sef′ ə lō sēl)
encephaloma (en sef′ ə lō′ mä)
oncology (on kol′ ō jē)
osteitis (os tē ī′ tis)
osteomalacia (os′ tē ō mä lā′ zhə)
pathologist (path ol′ ō jist)

endosteoma
   (en dos tē ō′ mä)
exogenous
   (eks oj′ ə nus)
histology (his tol′ ō jē)
hyperemesis (hī per em′ ə sis)
hypertrophy (hī per′ tro fē)
hypodermic (hī pō der′ mik)
intercostal (in ter kos′ t'l)
laryngitis (lair an jī′ tis)
lipoid (lip′ oid)
lipoma (lī pō′ mä)
morphology (mor fäl′ ō jē)
mucoid (myoo′ koid)
thyroidectomy
   (thī roy dek′ tō mē)
tracheotomy (trā kē ot′ ō mē)

Take a short break and then test yourself with the Unit 2 Self-Test,
next page.

Unit 2 Self-Test

Part 1

From the list on the right, select the correct meaning for each of the following terms. Write the letters in the space provided.

_____ 1. Osteomalacia	a. Overdevelopment
_____ 2. Intercostal	b. Study of microscopic tissues
_____ 3. Emesis	c. Surgical removal of cartilage
_____ 4. Adenoma	d. Between the ribs
_____ 5. Laryngotomy	e. Surgical repair of a joint
_____ 6. Lipoid	f. Softening of bone tissue
_____ 7. Cephalalgia	g. Herniation of brain tissue
_____ 8. Morphology	h. Tumor of glandular tissue
_____ 9. Carcinogenic	i. Headache
_____ 10. Encephalocele	j. Incision into the larynx
_____ 11. Arthroplasty	k. Pertainiing to producing cancer
_____ 12. Oncologist	l. Resembling fat
_____ 13. Hypertrophy	m. Vomiting, to vomit
_____ 14. Chondrectomy	n. Medical specialist dealing with tumors
_____ 15. Histology	o. The science of studying the structure of an organ

Part 2

Complete each of the medical terms on the right with the appropriate prefix and/or suffix:

1. Surgical removal of the thyroid gland   Thyroid _____

2. Inflammation of glandular tissue   Aden _____

3. Malignant tumor   Carcin _____

4. Excessive vomiting   _____ emesis

5. Resembling mucus   Muc _____

6. Tumor specialist   Onc _____

7. Making a new permanent opening into the colon   Col _____

8. Inflammation inside the head   _____ cephal _____

9. Tumor of fat tissue   _____ oma

10. Pertaining to the teeth   Dent _____

11. To breathe out   _____ hale

12. Pertaining to between the ribs   _____ cost _____

13. A tumor inside the bone canal   _____ oste _____

14. Medical condition resulting from an *under*active thyroid   _____ thyroid _____

15. Originating or produced completely outside of an organ or organism   _____ genous

ANSWERS

Part 1	Part 2
1. f.	1. Thyroidectomy
2. d.	2. Adenitis
3. m.	3. Carcinoma
4. h.	4. Hyperemesis
5. j.	5. Mucoid
6. l.	6. Oncologist
7. i.	7. Colostomy
8. o.	8. Encephalitis
9. k.	9. Lipoma

10. g.	10. Dental
11. e.	11. Exhale
12. n.	12. Intercostal
13. a.	13. Endosteoma
14. c.	14. Hypothyroidism
15. b.	15. Exogenous

3 Basic Anatomical Terms and Abnormal Conditions

In Unit 3 you will put together at least 50 new medical terms. You'll work with some new prefixes and suffixes and practice using those you covered in earlier units. Although this program doesn't attempt to teach anatomy of the human body, the language of medicine is all about the human body and what affects its parts. So, in this unit you'll bring anatomy and medicine together by focusing on a couple of anatomical areas and some abnormal conditions that affect them.

Mini-Glossary

abdomin/o (*abdomen*)

cephal/o (*head*)

chol/e (*bile, gall*)

cocc/i (*coccus*)

crani/o (*cranium, skull*)

cyst/o (*bladder, sac*)

dipl/o (*double*)

hydro (*water*)

lith/o (*stone, calculus*)

metr/o, meter (*measure*)

ot/o (*ear*)

pelv/i (*pelvis*)

phob/ia (*fear*)

py/o (*pus*)

rhin/o (*nose*)

staphyl/o (*grape*)

strept/o (*chain*)

therap/o (*treatment*)

thorac/o (*thorax*)

ab- (*away from*)

ad- (*toward*)

-ar (*pertaining to*)

-centesis (*puncture of a cavity*)

-genesis, gen/o (*produce, originate*)

-meter (*measuring instrument*)

-orrhea (*flow, discharge*)

Before you begin Unit 3, take the time to complete the Review Sheet for Unit 2. It will refresh your memory of the terms and word parts you studied. It may surprise you to find out how much you've learned. Try it (page 249).

1.
The prefix *ab-* means from or away from.

away from

Abnormal means ＿＿＿＿＿＿＿＿＿＿＿＿ normal.

2.

from or away from

The prefix ab- means ＿＿＿＿＿＿＿＿＿＿＿＿＿＿＿.

3.

wandering from (the
    normal course of
    events)

Ab/errant uses the prefix ab- before the English word for wandering. What do you think the term ab/errant means? ＿＿＿＿＿＿
＿＿＿＿＿＿＿＿＿＿＿＿＿＿＿＿＿＿＿＿＿.

4.

ab/errant
aberrant
ab er′ ant

Ab/errant is used in medicine to describe a structure that wanders from the normal. When some nerve fibers follow an unusual route, they form an ＿＿＿＿＿ / ＿＿＿＿＿＿＿＿＿ nerve.

5.

aberrant

Aberrant nerves wander from the normal nerve track. Blood vessels that follow an unusual path are called ＿＿＿＿＿＿＿＿＿ vessels.

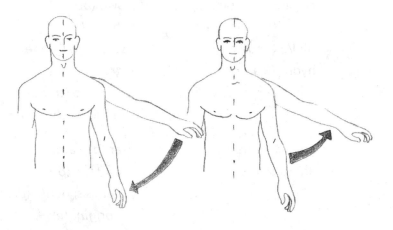

Figure 3.1   Adduction/Abduction

ab/duction
abduction
ab duk′ shun

6.
Ab/duct/ion means movement away from a midline. When the arm is raised from the side of the body,

_____ / _____ has occurred.
   away from   movement
   (midline)

abducted

7.
When children have been kidnapped and taken from their parents, they have been _____.

abducted

8.
Abduction can occur from any midline. When the fingers of the hand are spread apart, four fingers have been _____ from the midline of the hand.

ad/duction
adduction
ad duk′ shun

9.
On the other hand, *ad-* is a prefix meaning toward. Movement toward a midline is _____ / _____.

ab–
ad–

10.
The prefix meaning from or away from is _____. The prefix meaning toward, or toward the midline, is _____.

ad/<u>hesion</u>

11.
When two normally separate tissues join together, they adhere to each other like adhesive tape. Underline the part of the word that means sticking or joining: ad/hesion.

ad/hesion
adhesion
ad hē′ zhun

12.
Several years ago patients did not walk soon enough after surgery, which sometimes resulted in abnormal joining of tissues to each other. Write the word that means the abnormal joining and healing together of tissues: _____ / _____.

adhesions

13.
Now patients walk the day following an appendectomy. This has nearly eliminated _____.

14.

Review Exercise

Complete the following:

away from   The prefix ab– means _____ the midline.
toward   The prefix ad– means _____ the midline.

In your own words, explain the meaning of the following terms:

movement away from
  the midline   abduction _____.
sticking or joining
  together   adhesion _____.
a structure that wanders
  from the normal   aberrant _____.
a condition away from
  normal   abnormal _____.
movement toward a
  midline   adduction _____.

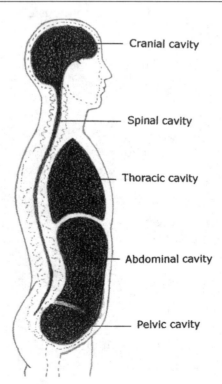

Cranial cavity

Spinal cavity

Thoracic cavity

Abdominal cavity

Pelvic cavity

Figure 3.2 The Great Cavities

The Great Cavities are closed cavities not open to the outside of
the body. Many of the body organs are suspended in these interval

chambers and provide cushions against shocks. The cavities allow body organs to assume various sizes and shapes. The *cranial cavity* and *spinal cavity* are continuous and house the brain and spinal cord. The *thoracic cavity* contains the lungs and major blood vessels and other structures. The *abdominal cavity* is where the stomach, liver, spleen, and intestines are found. The lower portion of the abdominal cavity is set apart as the *pelvic cavity*. Here's where the female reproductive organs, urinary bladder, and male ducts may be found.

Cranium (crani/o)   Thorax (thorac/o)
Abdomen (abdomino/o)   Pelvis (pelv/i)

Refer to the illustration above to help you complete many of the following frames.

belly
abdominal cavity
or abdomen
ab dō′ men
of
or pertaining to the
    abdomen, or
    abdominal cavity
	15.
	Abdomin/o is used to form words about the abdominal cavity or belly. When you see abdomin/o in a word, you think of the
	
	_____.
	
	Abdomin/al is an adjective that means _____
	_____.

abdomin/o/centesis abdominocentesis ab dom′ i nō sen tē′ sis	**16.** Abdomin/o/centesis means tapping or puncturing the abdomen to remove fluid. This is a surgical puncture of a cavity. The word for surgical puncture of the abdominal cavity is _____ / _____ / _____. abdomen puncture of a cavity
abdominocentesis	**17.** *Centesis,* or surgical puncture of a cavity, is a word in itself. Build a term meaning surgical puncture or tapping of the abdomen: _____.
abdominocentesis	**18.** When fluid has accumulated in the abdominal cavity, it can be drained off by a procedure called _____.
cardi/o/centesis cardiocentesis kär′ dē ō sen tē′ sis	**19.** Try this. The word for surgical puncture of a heart chamber is _____ / _____ / _____. heart puncture of a cavity

20.
Abdomin/o/cyst/ic means pertaining to the abdomen and urinary bladder. The word root for bladder is _____.

cyst

Cyst/o is used to form terms that refer to the _____.

bladder

To refer to the urinary bladder or any sac containing fluid, use some form of _____ / _____.

cyst/o

cyst/otomy
cystotomy

21.
The word for temporary incision into a bladder is

_____ / _____.
    bladder   incision into (temporary)

cyst/itis
cystitis
cyst/ectomy
cystectomy

Inflammation of a bladder is _____.

The word for surgical removal of a bladder is _____.

22.
Chances are good that by now you have figured out how word parts go together to create meaning. But let's review a simple rule and some examples.

Rule: About 90 percent of the time, the meaning of a term can be unscrambled by identifying its component parts in reverse.

For example,
  cyst means bladder;
  -itis means inflammation of.

inflammation of the
  bladder

Therefore cystitis means _____.

Dermat means skin;
-ologist means a specialist (one who studies).

one who studies the
  skin, or a skin
  specialist

Therefore dermatologist means _____
_____.

Abdomino means abdomen;
-centesis means surgical puncture of a cavity (to drain off fluid).

puncture of the
  abdominal cavity (to
  drain fluid)

Therefore abdominocentesis means _____
_____.

23.
Take a look at Illustration 3.2.

pertaining to the abdomen and thorax (bony cage forming the chest cavity)

The bony cage that forms the chest cavity is called the *thorax*. What does abdomin/o/thorac/ic mean? _____
_____
_____.

abdomin/o/thorac/ic
abdominothoracic
ab dom′ ɔ nō thō rā′ sik

24.
A word that means, literally, pertaining to the abdomen and chest cavity is _____ / _____ / _____.
                       abdomen   thorax   pertaining to

thorac/ic
thoracic
thō rā′ sik

25.
Thorac/o forms words about the thorax, or chest cavity. A word that means pertaining to the chest cavity is _____ / _____.
                                         thorax   pertaining to

thorac/otomy
thoracotomy
thōr ə kot′ ə mē

26.
Write a term meaning incision into the chest cavity:
_____ / _____.

thorac/o/centesis
thoracocentesis
thōr′ ə kō sen tē′ sis

27.
Write a term meaning surgical tapping of the chest cavity to remove fluids: _____ / _____ / _____.
                                thorax   puncture of

thorac/o/plast/y
thoracoplasty
thōr′ ə kō plas′ tē

28.
A word for the surgical repair of the chest cage is
_____ / _____ / <u>plast</u> / <u>y</u>.

cyst/o/plast/y
cystoplasty
sis′ tō plas′ tē

29.
Now write a word for surgical repair of a bladder:
_____ / _____ / _____ / _____.

30.
A hydro/cyst is a sac (or bladder) filled with watery fluid. *Hydro* is used in words to mean _____
_____.

water, fluid, or a watery fluid

31.

Go back to Illustration 3.2. The space inside the head is called

the cranial cavity _____.

head, including
   cranium and facial
   bones

Cranium means skull. Cephal/o is the combining form meaning _____

_____.

of or pertaining to
   the head

Therefore, cephalic means _____

_____.

32.

An increased amount of fluid in the head is called hydro/cephal/us. Both the fluid and the brain occupy the same space, called the

cranial cavity _____.

33.

hydro/cephal/us
hydrocephalus
hī′ drō sə fal′ us

A disease characterized by an enlarged head due to an increased amount of fluid in the cranial cavity is called

_____ / _____ / <u>us</u> .
      water   head

34.

Unless arrested, accumulation of watery fluid in the cranial cavity results in deformity of the skull, and brain damage may occur. This

hydrocephalus

condition is called _____.

35.

Hydro/phob/ia means having an abnormal fear of water. *Phobia*

abnormal fear

means _____.

36.

hydro/phob/ia
hydrophobia
hī drō fō′ bē ə

An abnormal fear of water is

_____ / _____ / _____ .
      water   abnormal fear

hydrophobia

Some parents are abnormally afraid to have their children swim or even ride in a boat. These parents suffer from _____.

37.

hydro/therapy
hydrotherapy
hī′ drō ther′ ə pē

Therapy means treatment. Treatment by means of water is

_____ / _____ .
      water   treatment

hydrotherapy

Swirling water baths are a form of _____.

38.
See Illustration 3.2 again, the bones of the pelvis form the pelvic cavity. A physician measures the size of a woman's pelvic cavity after she becomes pregnant. This procedure is called pelvi/metr/y.

pelvi

The word root for pelvic cavity is _____.

metr

The root for measurement is _____.

-y

The ending meaning a procedure is _____.

39.
To determine whether a woman has a pelvis large enough to avoid trouble during labor, a physician can measure the size of the pelvic cavity. This measurement is called _____.

pelvimetry
pel vim′ ə trē

40.
What do you think a pelvimeter is? _____
_____
_____.

a measuring device
    used for pelvimetry
    (or equivalent)

41.
When a physician measures the patient's pelvic cavity, the doctor is making a measurement called _____.

pelvimetry
pelvimeter
pel vim′ ə ter

The instrument used is a _____.

42.
Crani/o is used in terms referring to the cranial cavity or crani/um, or skull. Crani/o/plast/y means _____
_____.

surgical repair of the
    skull or cranium

43.
Write a medical term for each of the following:
a surgical procedure to excise part of the cranium,

crani/ectomy
craniectomy
krā nē ek′ tō mē

_____ / _____;
                skull   excision of

crani/otomy
craniotomy
krā nē ot′ ō mē

incision into the skull,

_____ / _____;
                cranium   incision into

crani/o/meter
craniometer

an instrument to measure the cranium,

_____ / _____ / _____.

of, or pertaining to, the
brain and skull
(cranium)

44.
The cerebrum occupies the cranial cavity. Thinking occurs in the
cerebrum (cerebr/o). What is the meaning of crani/o/cerebr/al?
_____
_____

cerebrum

45.
Have you ever been told to use your "gray matter"? Gray matter
controls thinking, feeling, and movement. The gray matter is the
largest part of the brain. What is it called? _____
cranium or cerebrum

cerebr/al
cerebral
ser ē′ brəl

46.
Write a term meaning of, or pertaining to, the gray matter of the
brain: _____ / _____.
            cerebrum   pertaining to

spin/al
spinal
spī′ nəl

47.
Cerebr/o/spin/al refers to the brain and spinal cord. What part
of the word means pertaining to the spinal cord?
_____ / _____.

cerebr/o/spin/al
cerebrospinal
ser ē brō spī′ nəl

48.
A puncture or tap to remove fluid from the space around the
cerebrum and spinal cord is called a spinal tap or
_____ / _____ / _____ / _____ puncture.
        cerebrum   spinal   pertaining to

49.
Review Exercise

SUGGESTED ANSWERS:
head   pelvis
bladder, sac   bony vault, skull
abdomen   chest cavity, rib cage
measurement   water, fluid

Using the suggested answers (only if you must), write the meaning
of each of the following:

pelvis, pelvic cavity
water, fluid
bladder, sac
head

pelv/i _____.
hydro– _____.
cyst/o _____.
cephal/o _____.

measurement, meter
bony chest cage, thorax
bony vault (brain), skull
abdomen, abdominal
    cavity

metr/o _____.
thorac/o _____.
crani/o _____.
abdomin/o _____.

50.
Try that again.

SUGGESTED ANSWERS:
-therapy	-otomy
-plasty	-metry
-ectomy	-centesis

Some suggestions:
(Yours may be
    different.)

Add a prefix or ending to each of the following combining forms and then explain the meaning of the term you created.

craniotomy

crani/o_____

pelvimetry

pelv/i _____

thoracoplasty

thorac/o _____

abdominocentesis

abdomin/o _____

cystectomy

cyst/o _____

hydrotherapy

hydro- _____

51.
Let's try something different. Coccus is a bacteria that causes disease. Cocc/i is the plural of cocc/us. When building terms about a whole family of bacteria called the cocci, we use the word root

cocc

_____.

(See Appendix B for more information on the formation of plurals.)

52.
Pneumonia is caused by the pneumococcus. From this term you know that the germ responsible for pneumonia belongs to the family of bacteria called _____ / _____ (plural).

cocc/i
kok′ sē

53.
There are three main types of a coccus bacteria:

dipl/o/cocc/i

cocci growing in pairs are
<u>dipl</u> / <u>o</u> / _____ / _____;

strept/o/cocc/i

cocci growing in twisted chains are
<u>strept</u> / <u>o</u> / _____ / _____;

staphyl/o/cocc/i

cocci growing in clusters are
<u>staphyl</u> / <u>o</u> / _____ / _____.

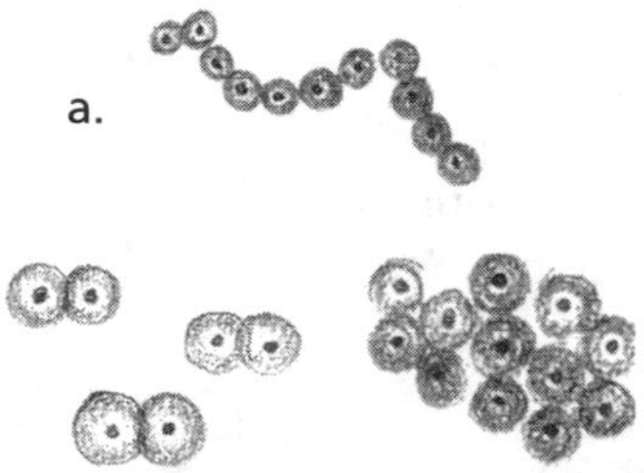

Figure 3.3   Cocci Bacteria   b.   c.

(a. strept)   (b. diplo)   (c. staphyl)

Bacteria (pl.) of the coccus family are round or spheroidal shaped single cell micro-organisms. Many types of cocci (pl.) exist and cause illness and infection in humans.

54.
Refer to the above frame for help. If you see a twisted chain of cocci when examining a slide under a microscope, you would say they were _____ / _____ / _____ / _____.

strept/o/cocc/i
strep′ tō kok sē

55.
Staphyle is the Greek word for bunch of grapes. If you should see a cluster of cocci when using a microscope, you would say they were _____ / _____ / _____ / _____.

staphyl/o/cocc/i
staphylococci
staf′ i lō kok′ sī

56.
The bacteria that cause carbuncles grow in clusters like bunches of grapes. Carbuncles are caused by _____ bacteria.

staphylococci

57.
Py/o is used for words involving pus. Genesis (gen/o) is from a Greek word meaning produce or originate. Py/o/gen/ic means _____.

pertaining to
producing pus

py/o/gen/ic
pyogenic

58.
Staphylococci produce pus; therefore, these cocci are
_____ / _____ / _____ / _____ bacteria.
         pus   producing

pyogenic

59.
Bacteria that contain or produce pus are referred to as
_____ bacteria.

pyogenic

60.
Boils are purulent (contain pus). This pus is formed by
_____ bacteria.
        pus-producing

discharge of pus

61.
The suffix -*orrhea* means flow or discharge. Py/orrhea means
_____.

py/orrhea
pyorrhea
pī ō rē′ ə

62.
The suffix –orrhea refers to any flow or discharge. A flow of pus is
called _____ / _____.
        pus   discharge

pyorrhea

63.
Pyorrhea alveolaris is a disease of the teeth and gums. The term that
tells you pus is being discharged is _____.

pyorrhea

64.
When pus flows from the salivary gland, the disease is called
_____ salivaris (of the salivary gland).

ear

65.
Ot/orrhea means a discharging ear; *ot-* is the word root for _____.

ot/orrhea
otorrhea
ō tō rē′ ə

66.
Ot/orrhea is both a symptom and a disease. No matter which is
meant, the word to use is _____ / _____.
                          ear   discharge

inflammation of the
(middle) ear

67.
Otorrhea may be a sign of ot/itis media (middle). Ot/itis media
means _____
_____.

otorrhea

This disease involves discharge, inflammation, pain, and deafness.
What's the term for discharge from the ear? _____

ot/algia
otalgia

68.
Otitis usually causes ear pain. Write the medical term for
_____ / _____.
    ear   pain

otalgia
ō tal′ jē ə

69.
Small children often complain of an earache. The medical term for
pain in the ear is _____.

nose

70.
Rhinorrhea means discharge from the nose. *Rhin/o* is used in terms
about the _____.

rhin/itis
rhinitis
rī nī′ tis

71.
Taking what is necessary from rhin/o, form a term meaning inflammation of the nose: _____ / _____.

rhin/orrhea
rhinorrhea

72.
When your head cold is accompanied by a "runny nose" the medical term for the symptom is _____ / _____.
                      nose   discharge

rhinorrhea

73.
Irritated or diseased sinuses in the head and face may discharge fluid
through the nose. This is a form of _____.

rhin/o/plasty
rhinoplasty

74.
Build a term that means surgical repair of the nose:
_____ / _____ / _____

rhin/otomy
rhinotomy

Form a word that means incision into the nose:
_____ / _____.

75.
Try these for a quick review.

SUGGESTED ANSWERS:

twisted, chainlike	double, paired
family of bacteria	producing, originating
pus	grape-like cluster
ear	nose

Using the suggestsions above (only if you must), write the meaning of each of the following:

family of bacteria   cocc/us, cocc/i _____

grape-like cluster   staphyl/o _____

pus   py/o _____

nose   rhin/o _____

double, paired   dipl/o _____

ear   ot/o _____

twisted, chain-like   strept/o _____

producing, originating   gen/o _____

76.
Try again. Here are some word parts and combining forms to help you build some familiar medical terms.

rhin/o	cocc/i
ot/o	py/o
-plasty	-orrhea
staphyl/o	gen/o
-algia	dipl/o

Put together a medical term that best defines each of the following descriptions:

diplococci   A family of coccus bacteria found growing in pairs _____.

pyogenic   Pertaining to producing pus, or pus-forming _____.

rhinorrhea   A runny discharge from the nose _____.

otalgia   Pain in the ear, earache _____.

    Bacteria of the coccus family growing in grape-like clusters

staphylococci   _____.

rhinoplasty   Surgical repair (reconstruction) of the nose _____.

77.
A rhin/o/lith is a calculus or stone in the nose. *Lith/o* is the combining form for _____.

calculus or stone

78.
Lithogenesis means producing or forming _____.

calculi (calculus) or
    stones

79.
Taking what is necessary from lith/o, build a word meaning an incision for the removal of a stone:

lith/otomy
lithotomy
lith ot′ə mē

_____ / _____.
      stone   incision into (for)

80.
Calculi or stones form in many places in the body. A chol/e/lith is a gallstone. Chole is the word for _____.

gall or bile

81.
One cause of gallbladder disease is the presence of a gallstone or

chole/lith
cholelith

_____ / _____.
      gall   stone

82.
No matter what its size or shape, irritation and blockage of the gallbladder can be caused by a bile or gallstone, called _____.

cholelith

83.
Gall is the fluid stored in the gallbladder. Cholecyst is a medical name for the _____.

gallbladder

84.
When gallstones cause inflammation of the gallbladder, this condition is called

chole/cyst/itis
cholecystitis
kō′ lē sis tī′ tis

_____ / _____ / _____.
      gall   bladder   inflammation

85.
Inflammation of the gallbladder is accompanied by pain and emesis. The condition is called _____.

cholecystitis

86.
Fatty foods like butter, cream, and whole milk contain fat and should be avoided by patients with an inflammatory condition of the gallbladder, or _____.

cholecystitis

chole/cyst/otomy
cholecystotomy
kō lē sis tot′ e mē
or
chole/lith/otomy
cholelithotomy
kō′ lē lith ot′ ə mē

87.
When a cholelith causes cholecystitis, one of two surgical procedures may solve the problem. One is an incision into the gallbladder
to remove stones, called a

_____ / _____ / _____
    gall   stone   incision into

or _____ / _____ / _____.
     gall   stone   incision into

chole/cyst/ectomy
cholecystectomy
kō′ lē sis tek′ tō mē

88.
More often, the presence of a gallstone calls for excision of the gallbladder, called

_____ / _____ / _____.
    gall   bladder   surgical removal

89.
It's time to review. From List B select the best meaning for each
term in List A. Write your choice in the space provided.

LIST A	LIST B
pelv/i _____	measure
lith/o _____	skull
chol/e _____	pus
py/o _____	pelvis
crani/o _____	head
cephal/o _____	gall, bile
metr/o _____	stone, calculus
rhin/o _____	chainlike
ot/o _____	double, pairs
strept/o _____	chest, thorax
staphyl/o _____	bladder, sac
dipl/o _____	nose
thorac/o _____	abdomen
cyst/o _____	grape-like
abdomin/o _____	ear

The words listed to the left of LIST A:

pelvis
stone, calculus
gall, bile
pus
skull
head
measure
nose
ear
chainlike
grapelike
double
chest
bladder, sac
abdomen

90.
Complete the following:

away from

The prefix ab- means _____ the midline.

toward

The prefix ad- means _____ the midline.

watery fluid, water

The prefix hydro- means _____.

91.

Select the best meaning for each of the following word parts.

treatment   therapy _____   surgical puncture
calculus, stone   lith _____   abnormal fear
discharge, flow   orrhea _____   calculus, stone
surgical puncture   centesis _____   treatment
abnormal fear   phobia _____   discharge, flow

92.

Each of the suffixes below means *of, or pertaining to* the word root to which it is attached. Write the meaning of each term.

	SUFFIXES	EXAMPLE	MEANING
of or pertaining to the duodenum	-al	duoden/al	_____
			_____
pertaining to the stomach	-ic	gastr/ic	_____
			_____
pertaining to the lumbar area (of the spine)	-ar	lumb/ar	_____
			_____
pertaining to the heart	-ac	cardi/ac	_____
			_____

93.

Here are more than 40 new medical terms you formed in Unit 3. Read them one at a time and pronounce each aloud. Better yet, ask a friend to say them aloud and you spell them.

aberrant (ab er′ ant)
abdominal (ab dom′ i nəl)
abdominocentesis
    (ab dom′ i nō sen tē′ sis)
abduction (ab duk′ shun)
adduction (ad duk′ shun)
cardiocentesis
    (kär′ dē ō sen tē′sis)
cephalic (cə fal′ ik)
cholecystectomy
    (kō′ lē sis tek′ tō mē)
cholecystitis (kō′ lē sis tī′ tis)
cholelithotomy
    (kō′ lē lith ot′ ə mē)
craniectomy (krā nē ek′ tō mē)
cranioplasty (krā′ nē ō plas′ tē)

craniotomy (krā nē ot′ ō mē)
cranium (krā′ nē um)
cystitis (sis tī′ tis)
cystocele (sis′ to sēl)
cystotomy (sis tot′ ə mē)
diplococci (dip′ lō kok′ sī)
hydrocephalus (hī′ drō sə fal′ us)
hydrophobia (hī′ drō fō′ bē ə)
hydrotherapy (hī′ drō ther′ ə pē)
lithogenesis (lith′ ō jen′ ə sis)
lithotomy (lith ot′ ō mē)
otalgia (ō tal′ jē a)
otitis (ō tī′ tis)
otorrhea (ō tō rē′ ə)
pelvic (pel′ vik)
pelvimetry (pel vim′ ə trē)

pyogenic (pī ō jen′ ik)
pyorrhea (pī ō rē′ ə)
rhinitis (rī nī′ tis)
rhinolith (rī′ nō lith)
rhinoplasty (rī′ nō plas tē)
rhinorrhea (rī nōr rē′ ə)
staphylococci (staf′ i lō kok′ sī)

streptococci (strep′ tō kok′ sī)
thoracic (thō rā′ sik)
thoracocentesis
   (thōr′ ə kō sen tē′ sis)
thoracoplasty (thōr′ ə kō plas′ tē)
thoracotomy (thōr ə kot′ ə mē)

Take the Unit 3 Self-Test before going on.

Unit 3 Self-Test

Part 1

From the list on the right, select the correct meaning for each of the following terms. Write the letter in the space provided.

_____ 1. Thoracocentesis

_____ 2. Cholelithotomy

_____ 3. Otorrhea

_____ 4. Cystotomy

_____ 5. Abdominalgia

_____ 6. Cranium

_____ 7. Cephalgia

_____ 8. Hydrophobia

_____ 9. Adduction

_____ 10. Streptococci

_____ 11. Pyogenic

_____ 12. Aberrant

_____ 13. Pelvic

_____ 14. Cholecystotomy

_____ 15. Rhinoplasty

a. Headache

b. Relating to the pelvis, pelvic cavity

c. Wandering or out of the normal place

d. Tapping or puncturing the chest cavity (thorax)

e. Movement toward the midline

f. Abnormal fear of water

g. Running or draining from the ear

h. Incision into the bladder

i. Producing pus

j. The bony vault surrounding the brain

k. Incision for the purpose of removing a gallstone

l. Commonly referred to as a "belly-ache"

m. Cocci bacteria that grow in chains

n. Surgical repair or restoration of the nose

o. Incision into the gallbladder

Part 2

Complete each of the medical terms on the right with the appropriate word root:

1. Herniation of a bladder   _____ cele

2. Tapping or puncturing of the heart chamber   _____ centesis

3. Surgical repair of the bony vault that encloses the brain   _____ plasty

4. Earache   _____ algia

5. Gallstone   _____ lith

6. Inflammation of the nose   _____ itis

7. Measurement of the pelvis   _____ metry

8. Relating to the thorax   _____ ic

9. Collection of fluid in the head   Hydro _____

10. Incision into the cranium   _____ otomy

11. Relating to the formation of pus   _____ genic

12. Surgical repair of the chest cage   _____ plasty

13. Instrument for measuring the pelvis   _____ meter

14. Relating to the abdomen   _____ al

15. Surgical removal of the gallbladder   _____

ANSWERS

Part 1	Part 2
1. d	1. Cystocele
2. k	2. Cardiocentesis
3. g	3. Cranioplasty
4. h	4. Otalgia
5. l	5. Cholelith
6. j	6. Rhinitis
7. a	7. Pelvimetry
8. f	8. Thoracic
9. e	9. Hydrocephalus

10. m	10. Craniotomy
11. i	11. Pyogenic
12. c	12. Thoracoplasty
13. b	13. Pelvimeter
14. o	14. Abdominal
15. n	15. Cholecystectomy

4 The Genitals and Urinary Tract

Unit 4 is a little longer than the previous ones. Again, you'll be working with roots, prefixes, and suffixes. You'll make more than 50 new medical terms and practice defining them. You'll work with anatomical terms and some medical conditions associated with these areas of the body. There are illustrations showing the anatomy of the urinary tract and genital organs of both male and female. Make these illustrations work for you. Bookmark the pages and refer to them often. Move slowly. When you encounter a difficult example, go back a frame or two and work through it again. Help yourself understand before moving on.

Mini-Glossary

angi/o (*vessel*)

arter/i/o (*artery*)

blast/o (*embryo*)

colp/o (*vagina*)

crypt/o (*hidden*)

fibr/o (*fiber*)

hem/o, hemat/o (*blood*)

hyster/o (*uterus*)

kinesi/o (*motion*)

lys/o (*destruction*)

men/o (*menses*)

my/o (*muscle*)

nephr/o (*kidney*)

neur/o (*nerve*)

o/o (*egg, ovum*)

oophor/o (*ovary*)

orchid/o (*testes*)

peps/o, peps/ia (*digestion*)

pne/o (*air, breathe*)

pyel/o (*pelvis of the kidney*)

salping/o (*fallopian tube*)

scler/o (*tough, hard*)

spermat/o (*sperm*)

ureter/o (*ureter*)

urethr/o (*urethra*)

ur/o (*urine*)

a-, an- (*without*)

brady- (*slow*)

dys- (*pain*)

-blast (*embryonic*)

-y, -ia (*noun ending*)

-orrhagia (*hemorrhage*)

tachy- (*fast*)

-orrhaphy (*suture*)

-pexy (*fixation*)

-ptosis (*drooping*)

-spasm (*twitching*)

-sperm (*sperm*)

Did you remember to complete the Unit 3 Review Sheet before beginning this new unit? Practice, practice, practice. It really works (page 251).

1.
Brady is used in words to mean slow.

slow

Brady/cardia means _____ heart action.

brady/cardia
bradycardia
brad ē kär′ dē ə

2.
The term for abnormally slow heart action is

_____ / _____.

3.
Kinesi- is used in words to mean movement or motion. Brady/

slowness of movement

kinesia means _____.

4.

pain on movement or
movement pain

Kinesi/algia means _____

_____.

5.

kinesi/algia
kinesialgia
kin ē′ sē al′ jē ə

When moving any sore or injured part of the body, pain occurs. Moving a broken arm can cause pain described as

_____ / _____.

6.

kinesialgia

After your first horseback ride, almost any movement causes a condition called _____.

7.

kinesi/ology
kinesiology
kin ē′ sē ol′ ə jē

The suffix *-ology* means study of. (Remember ologist?) The study of muscular movements is

_____ / _____.
          movement   study of

8.

Kinesi/ology is the study of movement. The study of muscular movement during exercise is known as the scientific field of

kinesiology

_____.

9.

The whole science of how the body moves is embraced in the field

kinesiology

of _____.

10.

abnormally slow movement

Brady/kinesia means _____

_____.

11.

Tachy- is used in words to show the opposite of slow. Thus

abnormally fast or rapid heart action

tachy/cardia means _____

_____.

tachy/cardia
tachycardia
tak ə kär′ dē ə

12.

Write the medical term for an abnormally fast heartbeat:

_____ / _____.

13.

Pne/o comes from the Greek word *pneia* (breathe). Pne/o anyplace

breathe or breathing

in a word means _____.

14.

When pne/o begins a word, the "p" is silent. When pne/o occurs later in a word, the "p" is pronounced; for example, when you pro-

will
brad ip nē′ ə
silent

nounce brady/pnea, you _____ pronounce the letter "p."
(will/will not)

In the term pneumonia, the "p" is _____.
(pronounced/silent)

15.

slow breathing

Brady/pnea means _____.

tachy/pnea
tachypnea
tak ip nē′ ə

A word for rapid breathing is _____ / _____.

16.

The rate of respiration (breathing) is controlled by the amount of carbon dioxide in the blood. Increased carbon dioxide speeds up

tachypnea

breathing and causes _____.

tachypnea

17.
Muscle exercise increases the amount of carbon dioxide in the blood. This speeds respiration and produces _____.

without breathing

18.
The prefix *a-* literally means without. Thus apnea means _____ _____.

apnea
ap′ nē ə

19.
A/pnea really means temporary cessation of breathing. If the failure to breathe were not temporary, death would result. Temporary cessation of breathing is referred to as _____.

apnea

20.
If the level of carbon dioxide in the blood falls very low, temporary cessation of breathing results. This is called _____.

bradypnea

21.
If breathing is merely very slow, it is called _____.

tachypnea
a–

22.
When breathing is abnormally fast, it is called _____.
The prefix meaning without is _____.

dys/pne/a
dyspnea
disp′ nē ə

23.
The prefix *dys-* means painful, bad, or difficult. Dys/troph/y literally means bad development. Write a word for difficult breathing: _____ / _____.

dys–

24.
Dys/men/orrhea means painful menstruation. The prefix for painful, bad, or difficult is _____.

poor or painful
    digestion

25.
Pepsis (peps/o) is the Greek word for digestion. Dys/peps/ia means _____.

dys/peps/ia
dyspepsia
dis pep′ sē ə

26.
Eating under tension may cause painful or poor digestion. This is called _____ / _____ / _____.

27.

dyspepsia

Contemplating the troubles of the world while eating is a good way to cause _____.

28.

Here's a quick review of what you just covered. From List B select the best meaning for each term in List A. Write your choice in the space provided.

	LIST A	LIST B
menses	men/o _____	digestion
digestion	peps/o _____	movement
breathe, breathing	pne/o _____	menses
movement	kinesi/o _____	breathe, breathing

29.
Try these.

	LIST A	LIST B
painful	dys- _____	very slow
very slow	brady- _____	painful
abnormally fast	tachy- _____	without, absence of
without, absence of	a- _____	abnormally fast

30.
Build a word for each of the following definitions using a prefix you just learned.

a/pnea	absence of breath _____ / _____
tachy/cardia	fast heartbeat _____ / _____
brady/kinesia	slow movement _____ / _____
dys/pepsia	painful digestion _____ / _____

Take a short break before beginning the next segment.

Refer to the table below to work through the next thirteen frames.

Some Combining Forms	
angi/o	vessel, blood & lymphatic
arteri/o	artery
fibr/o	fibrous, fiber
hem/o, hemat/o	blood
malac/o	soft, softened
lip/o	fat
my/o	muscle
neur/o	nerve or neuron
scler/o	hard

Some Suffixes	
-lysis	declining, dissolution
-spasm	twitch, twitching
-blast	germ or immature
-osis	condition of
-oma	tumor
-ia, -y	these endings make the term a noun

Table 1

neur/o/blast
neuroblast
nyoo′ ro blast

31.
An immature (germ) cell from which muscle tissue develops is a my/o/blast. A germ cell from which a nerve cell develops is a
_____ / _____ / _____.

angi/o/blast
angioblast
an′ jē ō blast

32.
A germ cell from which vessels develop is an
_____ / _____ / _____.

my/o/spasm
myospasm
mī′ ō spa zm

33.
A spasm of a nerve is a neur/o/spasm.

A spasm of a muscle is a
_____ / _____ / _____.

angi/o/spasm
angiospasm
an′ jē ō spa′ zm

A spasm of a vessel is an
_____ / _____ / _____.

angi/o/scler/osis
angiosclerosis
an′ jē ō sklə rō′ sis

34.
A (condition of) hardening of nerve tissue is neur/o/scler/osis. A hardening of a vessel is
_____ / _____ / _____ / _____.
   vessel   hardening   condition of

my/o/scler/osis
myosclerosis
mī′ ō sklə rō′ sis

A hardening of muscle tissue is

_____ / _____ / _____ / _____ .

35.
A tumor containing muscle and fibrous connective tissue is a my/o/fibr/oma. A tumor containing fibrous connective tissue and nerve tissue is a

_____ / _____ / _____ / _____ .

      nerve   fibrous tissue   tumor

neur/o/fibr/oma
neurofibroma
nyōō′ rō′ fī brō′ mä

angi/o/fibr/oma
angiofibroma
an′ jē ō fī brō′ mä

A vessel tumor containing fibrous connective tissue is a(n)

_____ / _____ / _____ / _____ .

neur/o/lys/is
neurolysis
nyōō rol′ ə sis

angi/o/lys/is
angiolysis
an jē ol′ i sis

36.
The destruction of muscle tissue is my/o/lys/is.

The destruction of nerve tissue is

_____ / _____ / _____ / _____ .

The destruction or breaking down of vessels is

_____ / _____ / _____ / _____ .

arteri/o/scler/osis
arteriosclerosis
ar ter′ ē ō skler ō′ sis

37.
Refer to the table only when you must. Arteri/o is used in words about the arteries. A word meaning hardening of the arteries is

_____ / _____ / _____ / _____ .

arteri/o/scler/osis
arteriosclerosis

a softened artery
arteriomalacia
ar ter′ ē ō mä lā′ zha

38.
Build a word meaning a hardened condition of the arteries:

_____ / _____ / _____ / _____ .

What do you think arteri/o/malac/ia means? _____

_____ .

arteri/o/spasm
arteriospasm
ar ter′ ē ō spa′ zm

lip/o/lys/is
lipolysis
lip ol′ i sis

39.
Build a word meaning arterial spasm:

_____ / _____ / _____ .

Dissolution (breakdown) of fat is called

_____ / _____ / _____ / _____ .

hem/angi/itis
hemangiitis
hē man′ jē ī tis

hem/o/lysis
hemolysis
hē mol′ ə sis
or another form is
   hemat/o/lysis
   hē mə tol′ ə sis

40.
Hem/o refers to blood. A tumor of a blood vessel is a
hem/angi/oma. (Note dropped o.) An inflammation of a
blood vessel is

_____ / _____ / _____.

Breaking down or dissolution of blood cells is

_____ / _____ / _____.

hemat/o/logy
hematology
hē mə tol′ ə jē

41.
Hemat/o also refers to blood. The study of blood is

_____ / _____ / _____.

hemat/o/logist
hematologist
hē mə tol′ ə jist

One who specializes in the science of blood is a

_____ / _____ / _____.

42.
Let's go over the new material again briefly. Match the best definition in List B with the word root in List A. Write your selection in
the space provided.

	LIST A	LIST B
artery	arteri/o _____	fat
fibrous connective tissue	fibr/o _____	muscle
blood	hem/o, hemat/o _____	artery
fat	lip/o _____	blood and lymph vessel
soften	malac/o _____	soften
muscle	my/o _____	harden
nerve	neur/o _____	fibrous connective tissue
harden	scler/o _____	blood
blood and lymph vessel	angi/o _____	nerve

Now match the best definition in List B with the suffix in List A.
Write the term.

	LIST A	LIST B
destruction of	–lysis _____	tumor
twitching	–spasm _____	science, or study of
tumor	–oma _____	condition of
inflammation of	–itis _____	twitching
germ cell (immature)	–blast _____	inflammation of
condition of	–osis _____	destruction of, dissolution
science, or study of	–ology _____	germ cell (immature)

43.
Build a word for each of the following definitions.

a condition of hardening of the arteries

arterio/scler/osis

_____ / _____ / _____

hemat/oma

blood tumor _____ / _____

angio/spasm

blood vessel spasm _____ / _____

myo/fibr/oma
  or fibromyoma

fibrous muscle tumor _____ / _____ / _____

neuro/blast

nerve tissue germ cell _____ / _____

lipo/lysis

breakdown of fat tissue _____ / _____

Take a break.

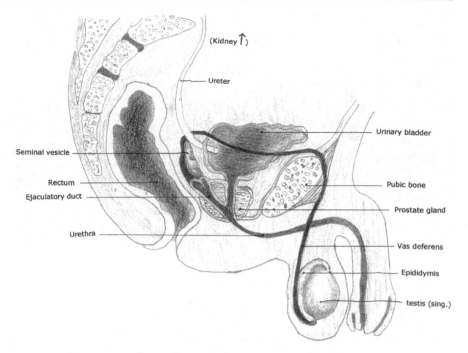

Figure 4.1   The Male Reproductive Organs (Midline Section)

The primary function of the male reproductive system is to produce *sperm cells* and deliver them to the female reproductive system for fertilization of the egg cells. The major organs of the male reproductive system are the paired *testes,* where sperm cells are produced. Surrounding the testis is a comma-shaped structure called the *epididymis.* Mature sperm cells are stored in the epididymis. The *vas deferens* is a long tube that conveys the mature sperm for ejaculation during copulation. It courses from the epididymis up into the body, over the pubic bone, curves to the left, passes the *urinary bladder,* curves again near the *ureter,* and passes downward. Here the vas joins with the duct leading from the *seminal vesicle* and forms the *ejaculatory duct.* The seminal vesicle is a small bladder-like structure that adds secretions to the sperm to form semen. The ejaculatory duct releases the semen and it enters the *urethra* as it exits the urinary bladder. The urethra is a 6 to 8 inch long tube in the male. It passes by the *prostate,* a chestnut-shaped gland surrounding the beginning of the urethra, and enters the penis, to deliver its contents for fertilization of the female egg cell.

Several accessory structures in the the diagram show their relationships to the reproductive organs. The ureter can be seen near the urinary bladder. It delivers urine from the kidney. The last portion of the large intestine is the *rectum,* and the end of the digestive tract is the *anus.*

sperm or spermatazoon (spermat/o)	ureter (ureter/o)
testis (orchid/o)	urethra (urethr/o)
prostate (prostat-, prostat/o)	

Review the illustration above, then refer to it as you work through the next 12 frames.

44.
The testes are organs that manufacture sperm, the male germ cell; that is, spermatozoa (plural) are formed in the _____.

testes (pl.)
testis (sing.)

45.
Orchid/algia means pain in a testicle or testis.

Orchid/ectomy means _____

_____.

excision of a testicle,
    testis

46.
Build a word meaning inflammation of a testicle,

_____ / _____;

incision into a testis, _____ / _____.

orchid/itis
orchiditis
or ki dī′ tis

orchid/otomy
orchidotomy
or kid ot′ ō mē

47.
A crypt/ic remark is one with a hidden meaning. A crypt/ic belief is obscure. The word root for hidden or obscure is

_____.

crypt
krıpt′

48.
Near the time of birth the testes of the fetus normally descend from the abdominal cavity into the scrotum. Sometimes this fails to happen, and the testes are not evident at birth. This condition of undescended testes is called

_____ / _____ / <u>ism</u> .
        hidden   testicle

crypt/orchid/ism
cryptorchidism
kript ôr′ kid ism

49.
When a testis is hidden in the abdominal cavity, the condition is called _____.

cryptorchidism

orchid/o/pexy

50.
An operation to repair cryptorchidism is called orchid/o/pexy.
Circle the part of the term that means to fix a testis in its place.

formation of
   spermatozoa, sperm,
   or male germ cells

51.
Sperma is the Greek word meaning seed.
Spermat/o is used in words about spermat/o/zoa or male germ
cells (sperm). Spermat/o/genesis means _____
_____.

spermat/o/lysis
spermatolysis
sperm′ ə tol′ i sis

spermat/o/blast
spermatoblast
sper mat′ ō blast

spermat/oid
spermatoid
sper′ mä toid

52.
Blast- means immature.
-Lysis means dissolution or destruction.

Give a word meaning the destruction of spermatozoa,

_____ / _____ / _____.

How about these:

an immature male cell, germ cell, sperm,

_____ / _____ / _____;

resembling sperm, _____ / _____.

53.
Summarize what you learned:

muscle
vessel
nerve

my/o   means _____,
angi/o   means _____,
neur/o   means _____.

54.
Again.

twitching, spasm
germ cell (immature)
hard, hardened
fibrous
destruction of

spasm   means _____,
blast/o   means _____,
scler/o   means _____,
fibr/o   means _____,
lysis   means _____.

55.
And these.

spermatozoa (sperm)	spermat/o	means	_____,
blood	hemat/o	means	_____,
blood	hem/o	means	_____,
formation of, or origination	genesis	means	_____.

Correct any definitions you may have missed; then cover the word roots, read the definitions you have written, and write the appropriate word root in the right-hand margin.

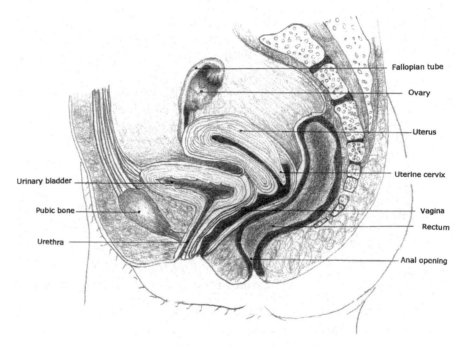

Figure 4.2 The Female Reproductive Organs (Midline Section)

The female reproductive system is responsible for producing female sex cells for potential union with male sperm cells. In addition, the female reproductive system nurtures the developing embryo and fetus for a nine-month period. The *ovaries* are the female reproductive organs in which egg cells are formed. An egg cell (*ovum*) is liberated into the *fallopian tube* and makes its way to the *uterus*. The uterus is a thick muscular organ that serves as a site for implantation of a fertilized ovum and nourishment of the embryo and fetus. A long narrow internal space leads from the uterus through a narrow neck called the *uterine cervix*. The cervix opens into the vagina. The *vagina* is a tubular organ approximately four inches in length. It receives the semen from the penis and transmits it to the uterus. It acts as a birth canal from the uterus to the outside for the newborn.

Other organs lie close to the female reproductive organs. Among these are the muscular *urinary bladder* and the *urethra*. The urethra is a short tube leading from the bladder which delivers urine to outside the body. The *rectum* is the last portion of the digestive organs and terminates at the *anus*.

ovary (oophor/o)	urinary bladder (cyst/o)
fallopian tube (salping/o)	urethra (urethr/o)
uterus (hyster/o)	vagina (colp/o)
ovum (o/o)	

Bookmark the illustration above and refer to it as you work through the next 20 frames.

56.
The Greek word for egg is *oon*. In scientific words, o/o (pronounce both o's) means egg or ovum. An o/o/blast is an immature _____ cell.

egg (a cell that will become an ovum)

57.
An ovum is discharged from the ovary. The combining form used in words referring to the ovary is *oophor/o*.

What does oophor/ectomy mean? _____
_____.

excision or surgical removal of the ovary

oophor/itis
oophoritis
ōō fôr ī′ tis

58.
Using what you need from oophor/o, build a word that means inflammation of an ovary: _____ / _____.

oophor/ectomy
oophorectomy
ōō fôr ek′ tō mē

59.
Oophor- is the root for ovary. Build a term for each of the following:
excision of an ovary, _____ / _____;

oophor/oma
oophoroma
ōō fôr ō′ ma

tumor of an ovary (ovarian tumor),
_____ / _____.

fixation (of)

60.
Oophor/o/pexy means fixation of a displaced ovary. *-Pexy* is a suffix meaning _____.

oophor/o/pexy
oophoropexy
ōō′ fôr ō pek′ sē

61.
When an ovary is displaced, a surgical procedure to fix it back in its normal place is called _____ / _____ / _____.

oophoropexy

62.
The surgical procedure to correct the position of a prolapsed (dropped or sagging) ovary is called an _____.

fallopian tube(s)

63.
Salping/o is used to build terms that refer to the fallopian tube(s). A salpingoscope is an instrument used to examine the _____.

salping/itis
salpingitis
sal pin jī′ tis

salping/ectomy
salpingectomy
sal pin jek′ tō mē

salping/ostomy
salpingostomy
sal pin gos′ tō mē

64.
Using what you need of salping/o, build a word meaning inflammation of a fallopian tube, _____ / _____;

excision of a fallopian tube,
_____ / _____;

a permanent opening into a fallopian tube,
_____ / _____.

game and good
   (pronounce them)

65.
In words built from laryng/o, pharyng/o, and salping/o, the "g" is pronounced as a hard "g" *when followed by an "o" or an "a."* The "g" in good is a hard "g." For example, in laryngalgia and salpingocele, the "g" of the word root is pronounced hard as in _____
_____.
(game/good) or (germ/giant)

hard (pronounce them)

66.
In laryngostomy, pharyngotomy, and salpingopexy, the "g" is followed by an "o" and is a _____
_____ sound.
(hard/soft)

"o" and "a"

67.
A hard "g" precedes the vowels _____ and _____.

germ and giant
(pronounce them)

68.
In words built from laryng/o, pharyng/o, and salping/o, the "g" is soft *when followed by an "e" or an "i"*; for example, in laryngectomy and salpingitis, the "g" is soft as in _____

_____.
(game/good) or (germ/giant)

soft (pronounce them)

"e" and "i"

69.
In salpingian, laryngitis, and pharyngectomy, the "g" is given a _____ sound because it
(soft/hard)

precedes the vowels _____ and _____.

laryngectomy
lar in jek′ tō mē
pharyngalgia
far ing gal′ jē a
pharyngitis
far in jī′ tis
salpingo-oophorectomy
   sal pin′ gō ōō fôr ek′
   tō mē

70.
Pronounce each of the following terms.

laryngectomy   pharyngitis
pharyngalgia   salpingo-oophorectomy

In each of the above terms circle the vowel that makes the "g" soft.

71.

In compound medical words, if two like vowels occur between word roots, they are separated by a hyphen. Use salpingo-oophorectomy as a model and build a word that means inflammation of the fallopian tube and ovary:
_____ / _____ / _____ / _____.

salping/o-/oophor/ itis
salpingo-oophoritis
sal′ pin gō ōō fôr ī′ tis

Use a hyphen between
   two like vowels when
   joining word roots

72.
Explain when a hyphen (-) is used in compound terms.
_____
_____
_____.

inflammation of the
   vagina

73.
Colp/o is used in words about the vagina. Colpitis means _____
_____.

vaginal spasm
colp/otomy
colpotomy
kôl pot′ ō mē

74.
A colp/o/spasm is a _____.

Incision into the vagina is a _____ / _____.

colp/o/plasty (you pronounce)

75.
Build a word meaning surgical repair of the vagina,

_____ / _____ / _____;

colp/o/scope
colposcope
kôl′ pō skōp

instrument for examining the vagina,

_____ / _____ / _____.

76.
Hyster/o is used to build words about the uterus. A hyster/ectomy is an excision, or surgical removal of, the _____.

uterus

77.
Write words for the following:

hysterotomy

an incision into the uterus, _____;

hysterospasm

a spasm of the uterus, _____;

hysteropexy

surgical fixation of the uterus, _____.

78.
Some terms are composed of many word roots plus a prefix and a suffix. These terms usually list the parts of the body in a special order.

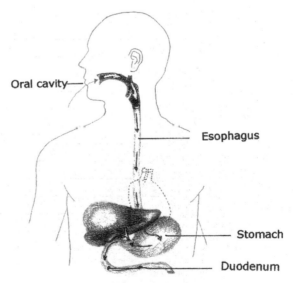

Figure 4.3   Path of EGD Examination

Take a look at Illustration 4.3 above. For example, when you swallow food it passes from the mouth to the esophagus to the stomach to the duodenum. So when a physician takes a look inside the digestive system with an endoscope the procedure is called

an endoscopic exam of the esophagus, stomach, and duodenum.

esophago / gastro / duoden / oscopy

Describe what the procedure EGD means. _____

_____.

79.
See Illustration 4.2, The Female Reproductive Organs. Examination of the female genital system begins at the vulva (external genitalia), then the vagina, and on to the uterus, fallopian tubes, and ovaries.

Follow the same order and build a word that means an operation to remove the uterus, fallopian tubes, and ovaries:

hystero/salpingo/ oophor/ectomy

_____

80.
Stop here and summarize what you've just covered. Match the best definition in List B with the word root in List A. Write your selection in the space provided.

	LIST A	LIST B
ovary	oophor/o _____	fallopian tubes
male germ cells	spermat/o _____	vagina
uterus	hyster/o _____	male germ cells
fallopian tubes	salping/o _____	egg, ovum
testicle	orchid/o _____	hidden
vagina	colp/o _____	testicle
egg, ovum	o/o _____	ovary
hidden	crypt _____	uterus
surgical fixation	-pexy _____	resembling
produce, originate	-genesis _____	twitching, spasm
resembling	-oid _____	suturing to repair
twitching, spasm	-spasm _____	produce, originate
germ cell, immature cell	-blast _____	germ cell, immature cell
suturing to repair	-orrhaphy _____	surgical fixation

81.
Build a word for each of the following:

colp/orrhaphy

suturing (to repair) the vagina, _____ / _____;

hystero/spasm

spasm of the uterus, _____ / _____;

orchido/pexy   fixation of the testis, _____ / _____;

salpingo/oophor/itis   inflammation of ovary and fallopian tube,
_____ / _____ / _____;

spermato/genesis   formation of spermatozoa,
_____ / _____;

spermato/blast   (immature) male germ cell,
_____ / _____.

82.
Now let's have some fun. Read each term and its meaning. Then study the accompanying illustrations.

Hernia is the protrusion of an organ, or part of an organ, through the wall of the cavity that normally contains it; a rupture.

Ptosis is the sinking down or sagging of an organ or part (from its normal position).

Anomaly is an irregularity. It is an organ or structure that is abnormal or contrary to the general rule.

Aneurysm is a localized abnormal dilation of a blood vessel, or ballooning out of the vessel at a weak point.

Write the correct term below each illustration:

Figure 4.4

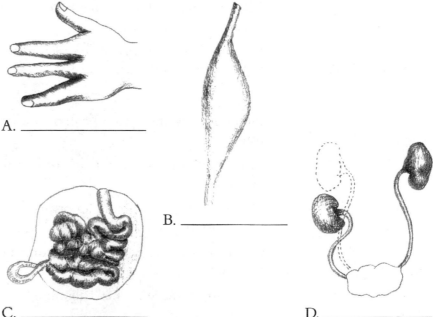

A. _____

B. _____

C. _____

D. _____

A. anomaly
B. aneurysm
C. hernia
D. ptosis

83.
Hyster/o/ptosis means prolapse (sagging) or sinking down of the uterus. Ptosis (pronounced tō′ sis) is a word that means _____ _____.

sinking down, prolapse, or sagging

84.
Upon examination, a physician may find that a patient's uterus has prolapsed or moved lower in the pelvic region. The medical term describing this condition is

hyster/o/ptosis

_____ / _____ / _____.

hyster/o/ptosis
hysteroptosis
his′ ter op tō′ sis

When uterine prolapse occurs, a surgeon may surgically fix the uterus back in its normal place. A hysteropexy would be done to correct or repair the condition known as

_____ / _____ / _____.

85.
From the terms provided, select one that best fits each definition.

anomaly   hernia   aneurysm   ptosis

hernia

Protrusion of an organ or part through the wall of the cavity in which it is normally enclosed. _____

ptosis

The prolapse, or sagging, of an organ or part from its normal position. _____

aneurysm

The abnormal ballooning out of a blood vessel at a weak point. _____

anomaly

Irregularity in structure of an organ or part; the structure is contrary to the general rule. _____

86.
Fill in the missing words to complete each of the following definitions.

normal

Ptosis is the sagging of an organ or part from its _____ position.

wall

Hernia is the protrusion of an organ or part through the _____ of a cavity that normally contains it.

Anomaly is an irregularity. It is an organ or structure that is contrary to the _____.

rule

Aneurysm is the abnormal ballooning out at a weak point in a

blood vessel

_____ _____.

87.
Complete each of the following descriptions by writing the form of the term that fits best.

anomalous (adjective)
anomaly is OK (noun)

An irregular organ or structure that is contrary to the general rule is said to be _____.

herniated (verb)

When an organ or part protrudes through the wall of the cavity that normally contains it, we say it has _____.

aneurysm (noun)

When a weak spot in the wall of the aorta (artery) balloons out, we call it an aortic _____.

nephr/o/ptosis

Nephr/o is used in words that refer to the kidney. If a kidney sags from its normal position, the medical condition is referred to as _____ / _____ / _____.

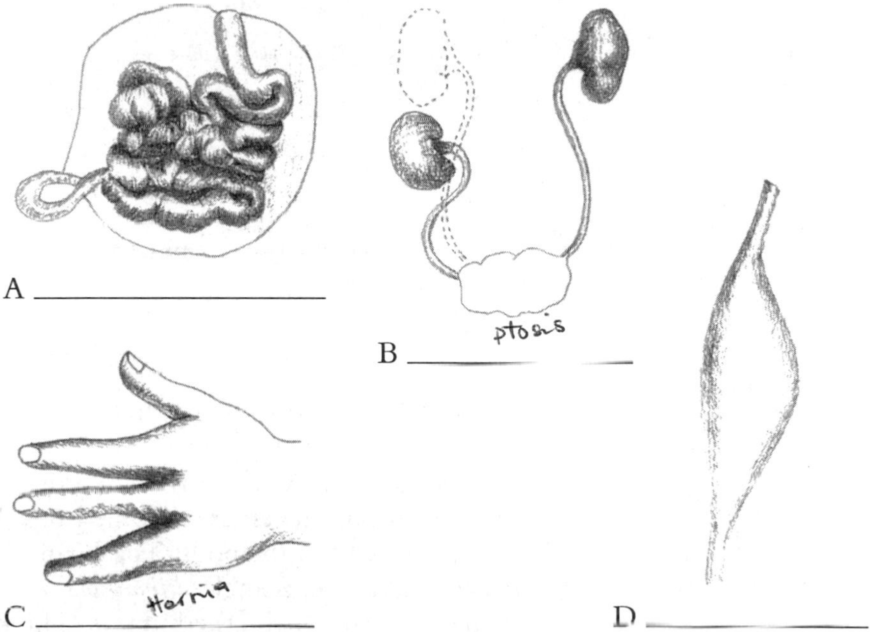

A. hernia
B. ptosis
C. anomaly
D. aneurysm

A _____

B _____
ptosis

C _____
Hernia

D _____

Figure 4.5 Label each illustration above.

88.
In your own words, write a brief definition for each of the following terms.

We suggest something like these:
aneurysm: an abnormal ballooning out of a blood vessel at a weak point.

aneurysm: _____
_____

anomaly: an organ or
structure that is
contrary to the rule.

anomaly: _____
_____
_____.

hernia: protrusion of an
organ or part through
the wall that normally
contains it.

hernia: _____
_____
_____.

ptosis: sagging of an
organ or part from its
normal location.

ptosis: _____
_____
_____.

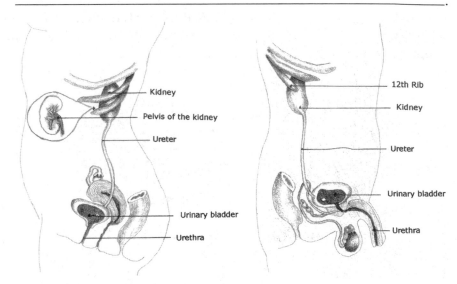

Figure 4.6   The Female Urinary Tract   **Figure 4.7**   The Male Urinary Tract

    The Urinary System involves elimination of waste, toxic prod-
ucts and surplus materials from the body. It also regulates the water
and salt content of the body. The Urinary Tract consists of paired
kidneys and *ureters,* a single *urinary bladder* and a urethra. The main
organs of excretion are the kidneys. The kidneys are bean-shaped
organs about the size of a fist. They are located on either side of the
spinal column and usually extend from the 12th rib. One kidney
touches the spleen and the other is slightly below the liver. A ureter
exits each kidney at the *renal pelvis.* This tube carries urine to the
main storage organ, the urinary bladder. The bladder is a hollow
muscular sac located in the midline at the floor of the pelvic cavity.
It can hold as much as 700–1000 ml of urine without injury. As it
distends, it rises into the abdominal cavity. The tube leading from

the bladder to the exterior is the *urethra*. This tube is about one and a half inches long in the female and about eight inches long in the male as it passes through the penis.

kidney (nephr/o)	renal pelvis (pyle/o)
bladder (cyst/o)	ureter (ureter/o)
urethra (urethr/o)	urine (ur/o)

89.
Let's go on to a new but related area of the body. Here is a brief summary of the functions of each part of the urinary tract.

kidney:	forms urine;
renal pelvis:	collects urine in the kidney;
ureter:	carries urine to the bladder;
bladder:	stores urine until voiding;
urethra:	discharges urine from the body.

90.
The urinary system is responsible for making urine from waste materials in the blood and carrying urine from the body. What is the word root for urine? _____. What is the combining form? _____.

ur
ur/o

91.
Pyel/o is the combining form that refers to the _____.

renal pelvis

92.
Taking what you need from the combining form for renal pelvis, form a term meaning inflammation of the renal pelvis,

_____ / _____;

surgical repair of the renal pelvis,

_____ / _____ / _____.

pyel/itis
pyelitis
pī ə lī′ tis

pyel/o/plasty
pyeloplasty
pī′ e lō plas tē

93.
Pyel/o/nephr/osis means _____ _____ _____.

abnormal condition of
the renal pelvis and
kidney

Form a term that means inflammation of the renal pelvis and kidney:

_____ / _____ / _____ / _____.

pyel/o/nephr/itis
pyelonephritis
pī′ lō nef rī′ tis

stone or calculus in the
   ureter

94.
Look at Illustrations 4.6 & 4.7. Ureter/o/lith means _____
_____.

ureter/o/lith/otomy
ureterolithotomy

Form a term that means incision into the ureter (for removal of a
stone):
_____ / _____ / _____ / _____.
        ureter   calculus   incision into

surgical repair of the
   ureter and renal
   pelvis

95.
Ureter/o/pyel/o/plasty means _____
_____
_____.

ureter/o/pyel/itis
ureteropyelitis
yo͞o rē′ ter ō pī ə lī′ tis

96.
Form a term meaning inflammation of the ureter and renal pelvis,
_____ / _____ / _____ / _____.

ureter/o/cyst/ostomy
ureterocystostomy
yo͞o rē′ ter ō sis tos′ tō
mē

97.
Form a term that means making a permanent opening between
the ureter and bladder,
_____ / _____ / _____ / _____.
        ureter   bladder   permanent opening

98.
Orrhaphy is not really a suffix, but again (for simplification) it can be
used as one. Orrhaphy means suturing or stitching (for the purpose
of repair, especially after trauma).

ureter/orrhaphy
ureterorrhaphy
yer rē ter ôr′ ə fē

Form a word meaning suturing of the ureter,
_____ / _____;

nephr/orrhaphy
nephrorrhaphy
nef rôr′ ə fē

suturing of a kidney,
_____ / _____;

cyst/orrhaphy
cystorrhaphy
sis tôr′ ə fē

suturing the bladder,
_____ / _____;

neur/orrhaphy
neurorrhaphy
nyo͞o rôr′ ə fē

suturing of a nerve,
_____ / _____.

99.

carries urine out of the body or removes urine from the bladder

Look back at Illustrations 4.6 & 4.7. What is the function of the urethra? _____

_____

_____.

urethr-

What is the word root for urethra? _____

suturing of the urethra (to repair)

Urethr/orrhaphy means _____

_____.

urethr/otomy
urethrotomy
yer ə throt′ ə mē

100.

Form a word that means incision into the urethra,

_____ / _____;

urethr/o/spasm
urethrospasm
yer rē′ thrō spasm

spasm of the urethra,

_____ / _____ / _____.

101.

Another complex word part is -orrhagia, which can be used as a suffix when it follows a word root. *Orrhagia* means bursting forth of blood (as in hemorrhage).

cyst/orrhagia
cystorrhagia
sis tō rä′ jē ə

Build a word that means bursting forth of blood from the bladder,

_____ / _____;

ureter/orrhagia
ureterorrhagia
yer rē′ ter ō rä′ jē ə

hemorrhage of the ureter,

_____ / _____.

ureter   bursting forth of blood

102.

Di/a is the combining form meaning pass through or secrete freely.

Define: (Use your Dictionary.)

diuresis _____.

How does the dictionary define these terms?

diuretic _____.

dialysis _____.

103.

Let's have a brief review. Select the correct word root or suffix from List B. Write your selection in the space provided in List A.

LIST A		LIST B
cyst/o–	stores urine until voiding _____	nephr/o–
aneurysm	ballooning-out vessel _____	pyel/o–
ureter/o–	carries urine to bladder _____	urethr/o–
anomaly	contrary to the rule, irregular _____	ur/o–
pyel/o–	collects urine in the kidney _____	ureter/o–
urethr/o–	discharges urine from body _____	cyst/o–
neur/o–	nerve _____	aneurysm
hernia	protrusion through cavity wall _____	anomaly
ur/o–	urine _____	hernia
nephr/o–	forms urine _____	neur/o–
–plasty	surgical repair (make new) _____	–lith
–ptosis	drooping, prolapse _____	–plasty
–pexy	fixing in place _____	–ptosis
–lith	stone, calculus _____	–orrhaphy
–orrhaphy	suturing to repair _____	–orrhagia
–ostomy	permanent opening _____	–ostomy
–orrhagia	hemorrhage _____	–spasm
–spasm	twitching, muscle cramp _____	–pexy

104.

Build a word for each of the following definitions.

diseased condition of renal pelvis and kidney

pyelo/nephr/osis ⟶ _____ / _____ / _____

incision to remove calculus from ureter

uretero/lith/otomy ⟶ _____ / _____ / _____

sagging of the kidney

nephro/ptosis ⟶ _____ / _____

the study of urine and the urinary system

ur/ology ⟶ _____ / _____

suturing, reconnection of the ureter

ureter/orrhaphy ⟶ _____ / _____

repair (make new) the kidney

nephro/plasty ⟶ _____ / _____

hemorrhage from the urinary bladder

cyst/orrhagia ⟶ _____ / _____

surgical fixing of the kidney in its place

nephro/pexy ⟶ _____ / _____

105.
Following are 50 of the medical terms you formed in Unit 4. Pronounce each one aloud and spell it on paper.

aneurysm (an′yo͞o rizm)

angioblast (an′ jē ō blast)

angiosclerosis
(an′ jē ō sklə rō′ sis)

anomaly (an om′ə lē)

apnea (ap′ nē ə)

arteriosclerosis
(ar ter′ ē ō skler ō′ sis)

arteriospasm
(ar ter′ ē ō spa′zm)

bradycardia (brad ē kär′ dē ə)

bradypnea (brad ip nē′ ə)

colporrhaphy (kôl pōr′ə fē)

colposcopy (kôl pōs′ kō pē)

cryptorchidism
(krip′ ôr kid ism)

cystorrhagia (sis tō rä jē ə)

dysmenorrhea
(dis′ men ōr rē′ ə)

dyspepsia (dis pep′sē ə)

dyspnea (disp′ nē ə)

hemangiitis (hē man jē ī′tis)

hematologist (hē mə tol′ ō jist)

hemolysis (hē mol′ ə sis)

hernia (her′ nē ə)

hysteropexy (his′ter ō peks′ ē)

hysterospasm (his′ter ō spa zm)

hysterotomy (his ter ot′ ō mē)

kinesialgia (kin ē′ sē al′ jē ə)

kinesiology (kin ē′ sē ol′ ə jē)

myosclerosis (mī ō skler ō′ sis)

myospasm (mī′ ō spa zm)

nephritis (nef rī′tis)

nephrolith (nef′rō lith)

nephromegaly (nef′rō meg ə lē)

nephroptosis (nef rop tō′ sis)

neurofibroma
(nyo͞o′ rō fī brō′ mä)

neurolysis (nyo͞o rol′ ə sis)

o-oblast (ō′ō blast)

oophoropexy (o͞o′ fôr ō pek′ sē)

orchidotomy (or kid ot′ ō mē)

pyelitis (pī ə lī′ tis)

pyeloplasty (pī′ ə lō plas tē)

salpingectomy
(sal pin jek′ tō mē)

salpingo-oophorectomy
(sal pin′ gō o͞o fôr ek′ tō mē)

salpingoscopy (sal pin gos′ kō pē)

spermatoblast (sper mat′ ō blast)

spermatoid (sper′ ma toid)

tachycardia (tak ə kär′ dē ə)

tachypnea (tak ip nē′ ə)

ureterolithotomy
(yer rē′ ter ō lith ot′ ō mē)

ureterorrhaphy
(yer rē ter ôr′ ə fē)

ureterotomy (yer ē ter ot′ə mē)

urethralgia (yer ə thral′ jē ə)

urethrotomy (yer e throt′ ə mē)

Complete the Unit 4 Self-Test before going to the next unit.

Unit 4 Self-Test

Part 1

From the list on the right, select the correct meaning for each of the following terms:

_____ 1. Urethrospasm

_____ 2. Spermatoid

_____ 3. Nephroptosis

_____ 4. Anomaly

_____ 5. Oophoropexy

_____ 6. Bradypnea

_____ 7. Angioblast

_____ 8. Ureterotomy

_____ 9. Angiosclerosis

_____ 10. Hysterotomy

_____ 11. Myospasm

_____ 12. Dyspepsia

_____ 13. Hemolysis

_____ 14. Kinesiology

_____ 15. Aneurysm

a. The study (or science) of motion

b. A condition of hardening of vessels

c. Spasm of the urethra

d. Destruction of blood (cells)

e. Abnormally slow breathing

f. Surgical fixation of the ovary in its place

g. Tumor of nerve and fibrous tissue

h. Muscle spasm

i. Structure contrary to the rule

j. Resembling sperm

k. Abnormally enlarged kidney

l. Ballooning out of blood vessel

m. Painful menstruation (cramps)

n. Vessel germ cell

o. Kidney out of its normal place (dropped kidney)

p. Incision into the uterus (cesarean section)

q. Painful digestion (heartburn)

r. Incision into the ureter

Part 2

Complete each of the medical terms on the right with the appropriate missing part:

1. A condition of hardening of muscle   _____ sclerosis

2. Kidney stone   Nephro _____

3. Abnormally fast breathing   Tachy _____

4. Painful menstruation   _____ menorrhea

5. Spasm of the uterus   _____ spasm

6. Cessation of menses   A _____

7. Hemorrhage (bleeding) from the bladder   _____ orrhagia

8. Surgical removal of the ovary   _____ ectomy

9. Incision into the ureter (for the purpose of removing a stone)   _____ lithotomy

10. Surgical removal of the fallopian tube   _____ ectomy

11. Drooping of an organ   P _____

12. Pain due to motion   _____ algia

13. Spasm of the vessels   _____ spasm

14. Protrusion of an organ through a cavity wall   H _____

15. Incision into the urethra   _____ otomy

ANSWERS

Part 1	Part 2
1. c	1. Myosclerosis
2. j	2. Nephrolith
3. o	3. Tachypnea
4. i	4. Dysmenorrhea
5. f	5. Hysterospasm
6. e	6. Amenorrhea
7. n	7. Cystorrhagia
8. r	8. Oophorectomy
9. b	9. Ureterolithotomy

10. p	10. Salpingectomy
11. h	11. Ptosis
12. q	12. Kinesialgia
13. d	13. Angiospasm
14. a	14. Hernia
15. l	15. Urethrotomy

<u>5</u> The Gastrointestinal Tract

In Unit 5 you'll make more than 50 new medical terms. Most of the learning material focuses on terms relating to the gastrointestinal tract. Two illustrations provide information you'll need as you work through the learning sequences and exercises. Be sure to bookmark those illustrations and keep them handy. Use them often.

Mini-Glossary

cheil/o (lip, lips)

col/o (colon)

dent/o (teeth)

esophag/o (esophagus)

gingiv/o (gums)

gloss/o (tongue)

hepat/o (liver)

pancreat/o (pancreas)

proct/o (anus and rectum)

rect/o (rectum)

stomat/o (mouth)

-clysis (irrigation)

-ectasia (dilation, stretching)

-scope, -scopy (look, examine)

-toxin (poison)

Take a few minutes to complete the Review Sheet for Unit 4 before you begin Unit 5.

1.
You're going to begin this section with a review of suffixes you have already studied and used.

Write the meaning of each of the following:

of, or pertaining to	–ic, –as, –ar _____
surgical repair, make new, restore	–plasty _____
inflammation of	–itis _____
twitching, cramping	–spasm _____
pain, ache	–algia _____
under, beneath	–hypo _____
excessive, too much	–hyper _____
surgical excision of	–ectomy _____
incision into	–otomy _____
bursting forth, hemorrhage	–orrhagia _____
a noun ending meaning condition, condition of	–a, –ia _____
abnormal condition, diseased condition	–osis _____

2.
This time, write the suffix that satisfies each of the definitions given. Then go back to the last frame to check your answers.

MEANING	SUFFIX
pain, ache	_____
excessive, too much	_____
surgical incision into	_____
inflammation of	_____
under, beneath	_____
twitching, cramping	_____
surgical excision of	_____
bursting forth, hemorrhage	_____
of, or pertaining to	_____
an ending meaning condition	_____
abnormal (diseased) condition	_____

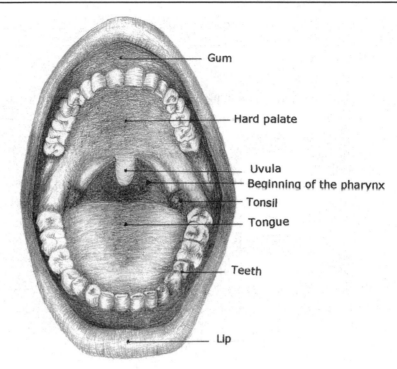

Figure 5.1 The Oral Cavity

The digestive tract begins at the mouth, the oral cavity. The human mouth is concerned with vocalization as well as mastication and swallowing. The anterior portion includes lips, teeth, gums, a muscular tongue, related muscles, salivary glands, a bony palate, and muscles of the cheek wall. All are concerned with wetting, macerating and pulverizing ingested material. The posterior portion of the oral cavity includes the soft palate, tongue, tonsils, and tastebuds.

mouth (stomat/o)	lip (cheil/o)
tongue (gloss/o)	gum (gingiv/o)
	tooth (dent/o)

3.

stomat	The word root for mouth is _____.
stomat/o	The combining form is _____ / _____.

4.

inflammation of the mouth	Stomat/itis means _____.

surgical repair or reconstruction of the mouth	Stomat/o/plast/y means _____
	_____.
stomat/algia	5.
stomatalgia	Using the word root for mouth, form a word meaning painful
stō mä tal′ jē ə	mouth, _____ / _____;
stomat/orrhagia	
stomatorrhagia	hemorrhage of the mouth,
stō mat′ ō rä′ jē ə	_____ / _____.
	mouth hemorrhage
	6.
	Refer to Illustration 5.1.
painful tongue	Gloss/algia means _____.
excision of the tongue	Gloss/ectomy means _____.
spasm or twitching of the tongue	Gloss/o/spasm means _____
	_____.
gloss/itis	7.
glossitis	Using the word root, build a term meaning inflammation of the
glos ī′ tis	tongue, _____ / _____;
gloss/al	
glossal	
glos′ əl	pertaining to the tongue, _____ / _____
	8.
hypo/gloss/al	What word would you use to describe a medication that is adminis-
hypoglossal	tered under the tongue?
hī′ pō glos′ əl	_____ / _____ / _____
	under tongue pertaining to
	9.
cheil	Go back to Illustration 5.1. The word root for lip is _____.
cheil/o	The combining form for lip is _____ / _____.
kē′ lō	
	10.
inflammation of the lips	Cheil/itis means _____
	_____.
plastic surgery of the lips	Cheil/o/plast/y means _____
	_____.

cheil/otomy
cheilotomy
kē lot′ ō mē

cheil/osis
cheilosis
kē lō′ sis

11.
Build a term meaning incision into the lips,
_____ / _____;

abnormal condition or diseased condition of the lips,
_____ / _____.

cheil/o/stomat/o/plasty
cheilostomatoplasty
kē′ lō stō mat′ ō plas tē

12.
Now, build a term meaning plastic surgery of the lips and mouth
_____ / ____ / _____ / ____ /_____.
　　lip　　　　　　　　　mouth　　　　　　　　　repair

gingiv/o
of or pertaining to gums

13.
The combining form for gums is _____ / _____.
Gingival means _____.

gingiv/itis
gingivitis
jin ji vī′ tis

gingiv/algia
gingivalgia
jin ji val′ jē ə

gingiv/ectomy
gingivectomy
jin ji vek′ tə mē

gingiv/o/gloss/itis
gingivoglossitis
jin′ ji vō glos ī′ tis

14.
Build a term meaning inflammation of the gums,
_____ / _____;

painful gums,
_____ / _____;

excision of gum tissue,
_____ / _____;

inflammation of the gums and tongue,
_____ / ____ / _____ / _____.

15.
Here's a quick review. Without referring to the tables, write a
meaning for each of the following.

inflammation of the
　　gums
surgical excision of
　　the tongue
toothache
plastic surgery, repair of
　　the lips
hemorrhage of the
　　mouth

gingivitis _____

glossectomy _____

dentalgia _____

cheiloplasty _____

stomatorrhagia _____

16.
Using the suggested word roots, make a medical term that fits each definition below.

Some suggested root words

stomat–
cheil–
gingiv–
gloss–
dent–

glossitis   inflammation of the tongue _____
cheilosis   abnormal, diseased condition of the lips _____
dentalgia   toothache _____
stomatoplasty   plastic surgery, repair of the mouth _____
gingivectomy   surgical excision of gum tissue _____

Take a break. You deserve it.

17.
Again, you will use many suffixes you are already familiar with. Here's an opportunity to refresh your memory. See how many you can correctly define. Write your answers in the space provided.

puncture of cavity, to   –centesis _____
   withdraw fluid
incision into   –otomy _____
form a new (permanent)   –ostomy _____
   opening
study of   –ology _____
surgical fixation of a   –pexy _____
   part in its normal
   place
hernia, herniation   –cele _____
calculus, stone   –lith _____
large, enlarged   –megaly _____

18.
Now, complete Table 3 below. You will use it in the next few frames. Write the suffix that satisfies the definition given. Check your answers in the last frame.

Table 3

Meaning	Suffix
calculus, stone	-_____
surgical fixation of a part in place	-_____
incision into	-_____
study of	-_____
hernia, herniation	-_____
large, enlarged	-_____
form a new opening (permanent)	-_____
puncture a cavity and draw fluid	-_____

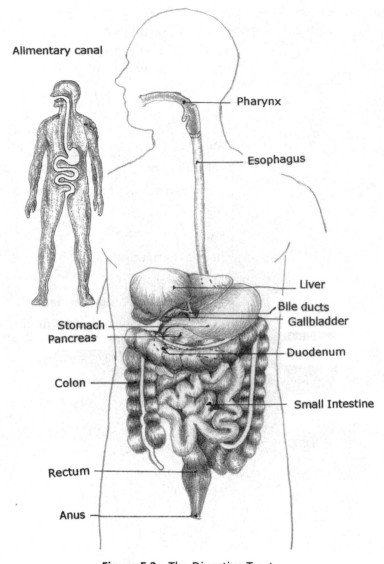

Figure 5.2   The Digestive Tract

The function of the digestive system is to break down large food particles into smaller ones that can pass across the membranes of cells and be absorbed. The Digestive Tract, also known as the *alimentary canal* consists of a single long tube extending from mouth to anus and opened to the exterior at each end. The canal begins with the oral cavity. Here the teeth pulverize ingested food. Meanwhile it is softened and partly digested by salivary gland secretions. The tongue aids in mechanical manipulation of the food and literally flips the food into the fibromuscular *pharynx* during swallowing. The *esophagus* moves the food bolus along to the pouch-like *stomach* by peristaltic muscular contractions. Here the food mixes with acid and protein-digesting enzymes and is retained until digested further. Passing from the stomach, the food enters the first part of the small intestine called the *duodenum.* Liver-produced bile, stored in the *gallbladder,* is discharged into the duodenum by *bile ducts.* Digestive enzymes from the *pancreas* enter the duodenum as well. The food bolus continues through the highly coiled 20-foot-long *small intestine.* A great portion of the abdominal cavity is taken up by the many folds and twists of this organ. Small molecular nutrients are extracted and absorbed by cells lining the intestine. These nutrients absorbed throughout the tract are transferred to capillaries and transported to the *liver* by the hepatic portal system for processing and distribution to the body's cells. The *colon* or large intestine can be seen ascending along the anatomical right side, passing across the midline then turning and descending along the left. This organ is mainly concerned with absorption of water, minerals, and certain vitamins. The non-nutritive residue of the ingested food is compacted and moved through the *rectum* and *anal canal* to the outside.

liver (hepat/o)	stomach (gastr/o)
pharynx (pharyng/o)	gallbladder (cholecyst/o)
esophagus (esophag/o)	duodenum (duoden/o)
intestine (enter/o)	colon (col/o)
rectum and anus (proct/o)	pancreas (pancreat/o)
rectum (rect/o)	anus (an/o)

19.

stomach hemorrhage   Here are some easy ones. Gastr/orrhagia means _____

inflammation of the   Gastritis means _____
    stomach   _____

of, or pertaining to the   Gastric means _____
    stomach   _____

20.

Here are some new suffixes.

-ectasia means dilation, stretching, or expansion
-clysis means irrigation, or washing out
-toxin means poison, or poisoning

Use Illustration 5.2 and write a meaning for the following medical terms.

poisoning of the small   enter/o/toxin _____
    intestine   _____

stretching, dilation of   enter/ectasia _____
    the small intestine   _____

irrigation, washing out   enter/o/clysis _____
    of the small intestine _____

21.

washing, irrigation of   What do you think col/o/clysis means? _____
    the colon   _____

dilation, stretching, or   What does gastr/ectasia mean? _____
    expanding of the   _____
    stomach

22.

Use Illustration 5.2 as you need to, and try these.

a surgical procedure to   col/o/pexy means _____
    fix the colon in its   _____
    normal place

herniation of the small   enter/o/cele means _____
    intestine   _____

a surgical procedure   col/ostomy means _____
    to make a new   _____
    (permanent) opening
    into the colon

gastr/o/enter/ostomy
gastroenterostomy
gas' trō en ter os' tō mē

23.
Form a term describing a surgical procedure that forms a new opening between the stomach and small intestine,

_____ / _____ / _____ / _____ ;

gastr/o/enter/ic
gastroenteric
gas' trō en ter' ik

pertaining to the stomach and small intestine,

_____ / _____ / _____ / _____ .

enter/o/clysis
enteroclysis
en ter ok' li sis

24.
Refer to Illustration 5.2 again. Build a term meaning washing or irrigation of the small intestine,

_____ / _____ / _____ ;

enter/ectasia
enterectasia
en' ter ek tā' jē ə

dilation of the small intestine,

_____ / _____ .

25.
What do the following terms mean?

poisoning of the small intestine

Enter/o/toxin _____

_____ .

puncture of the small intestine, draw fluid

Enter/o/centesis _____

_____ .

Enter/o/cele _____

intestinal hernia

_____ .

26.
Try these.

pertaining to the colon or large intestine

Col/ic _____

_____ .

puncture of the colon, draw fluid

Col/o/centesis _____

_____ .

making a new opening into the colon (permanent)

Col/ostomy _____

_____ .

col/o/pexy
colopexy
kō' lō pek sē

27.
Build a term meaning surgical fixation of the colon,

_____ / _____ / _____ ;

col/o/clysis
coloclysis
kō lok′ li sis

washing or irrigation of the colon,
_____ / _____ / _____;

col/itis
colitis
kō lī′ tis

inflammation of the colon, _____ / _____.

28.
Refer to Illustration 5.2 again. The combining form for rectum is

rect/o

_____ / _____.

What do each of the following mean?

pertaining to the
    rectum

Rect/al _____
_____.

a rectal hernia

Rect/o/cele _____
_____.

washing or irrigation of
    the rectum (enema)

Rect/o/clysis _____
_____.

rect/o/colitis
rectocolitis
rek′ tō kō li′ tis

29.
Build a word meaning inflammation of the rectum and colon,
_____ / _____ / _____;

rect/o/cyst/otomy
rectocystotomy
rek′ tō sis tot′ ə mē

incision of the bladder through the rectum,
_____ / _____ / _____ / _____.
    rectum   bladder   incision into

specializes in diseases of
    the anus and rectum

30.
Proctology is the study of diseases of the anus and rectum. A
proct/o/log/ist is one who _____
_____.

proct/o/clysis
proctoclysis (enema)

prok tok′ li sis

31.
Build a word meaning washing or irrigation of anus and rectum,
_____ / _____ / _____;

Pronounce that one several times.

instrument for
    examining the anus
    and rectum
    prok′ tə skōp

32.
Write a meaning for each of the following:

proct/o/scope _____
_____.

examination of the anus and rectum prok tos' kō pē	proct/o/scopy _____ _____.
	33. Back to Illustration 5.2. What is the combining form for liver?
hepat/o	_____.
pertaining to the liver	Hepat/ic means _____.
an abnormal condition of enlargement of the liver	Hepatomegaly means _____ _____.
hepat/o/scop/y hepatoscopy hep ə tos' kō pē	34. Build a word meaning inspection (examination) of the liver, _____ / _____ / _____ / _____;
hepat/otomy hepatotomy hep ə tot' ō mē	incision into the liver, _____ / _____;
hepat/itis hepatitis hep ə tī' tis	inflammation of the liver, _____ / _____.
	35. Here's another new term. Pancreat/ic means _____
pertaining to the pancreas	_____.
	Underline the part of the term that means dissolution or destruction.
pancreat/o/<u>lysis</u>	Pancreat/o/lys/is
pancreat/o/lith pancreatolith pan krē at' ə lith	36. Build a word meaning a stone or calculus in the pancreas, _____ / _____ / _____; pancreas stone
pancreat/itis pancreatitis pan krē a tī' tis	inflammation of the pancreas, _____ / _____;
pancreat/ectomy pancreatectomy pan krē a tek' tō mē	excision of part or all of the pancreas, _____ / _____;
pancreat/otomy pancreatotomy pan krē a tot' ə mē	incision into the pancreas, _____ / _____.

esophag/o/duoden/
    ostomy
esophagoduodenostomy
ē sof′ ə gō doo′ ō den
    os′ tō mē

37.
When an entire gastrectomy is performed, a new connection (opening) is formed between the esophagus and duodenum. This is called an _____ / _____ / _____ / _____.

(Note: Remember to name the anatomical parts in the order in which food passes through them.)

38.
As you rewrite each of the following, analyze it (make your own diagonal divisions) and pronounce it to yourself:

gastr/o/enter/o/col/
    ostomy

gastroenterocolostomy,

_____;

esophag/o/gastr/
    ostomy

esophagogastrostomy,

_____;

enter/o/chol/e/cyst/
    ostomy

enterocholecystostomy,

_____.

39.
Try it again:

Proctectasia,

proct/ectasia

_____;

duoden/o/chol/e/cyst/
    ostomy

duodenocholecystostomy,

_____;

esophag/o/gastr/o/
    scopy

esophagogastroscopy,

_____.

40.
Let's review what you just covered. Using the suggested answers, write the meaning of each of the following terms.

SUGGESTED ANSWERS:

colon	lips	rectum
duodenum	liver	anus and rectum
esophagus	mouth	small intestine
gums	pancreas	tongue
stomach		

rectum   rect/o _____
colon   col/o _____
pancreas   pancreat/o _____

rectum and anus	proct/o _____
lips	cheil/o _____
mouth	stomat/o _____
small intestine	enter/o _____
esophagus	esophag/o _____
gums	gingiv/o _____
tongue	gloss/o _____
liver	hepat/o _____
duodenum	duoden/o _____
stomach	gastr/o _____

41.
Try these.

SUGGESTED ANSWERS
make a new opening   stretching
poison   irrigation
look, examine

irrigation	–clysis _____
look, examine	–scope, –scopy _____
make a new opening	–ostomy _____
stretching	–ectasia _____
poison	–toxin _____

42.
In your own words, write the meaning of each of the following medical terms.

Here's what we suggest:

a new opening between the esophagus and duodenum

esophag/o/duoden/ostomy
_____
_____

inspection of the anus and rectum (with an instrument)

proct/oscopy
_____
_____

plastic surgery of the lips

cheil/o/plasty
_____
_____

stretching of the esophagus

esophag/o/ectasia
_____
_____

irrigation of the anus and rectum (and lower colon; enema)	proct/o/clysis
	_____
	_____
pain of the stomach and intestine	gastr/o/enter/algia
	_____
	_____
incision into the pancreas	pancreat/otomy
	_____
	_____
tumor of the mouth	stomat/oma
	_____
	_____
spasm of the tongue	gloss/o/spasm
	_____
	_____

43.

Here are 25 medical terms for practicing your pronunciation. Say the term aloud and then say what it means. Then take the Unit 5 Self-Test.

cheilitis (kē lī′ tis)
cheiloplasty (kē′ lō plas tē)
colic (kol′ ik)
colitis (kō lī′ tis)
colostomy (kō los′ tō mē)
dentalgia (den tal′ jē ə)
enterocele (en′ ter ō sēl)
enteroclysis (en ter ok′ li sis)
enterotoxin (en′ ter ō tox in)
esophagogastroscopy
    (ē sof′ ə gō gas tros′ kō pē)
gastrectasia (gas trek tā′ zhə)
gastrorrhagia (gas′ trō rä′ jē ə)
gingivectomy
    (jin ji vek′ tō mē)

gingivoglossitis
    (jin′ ji vō glos ī′ tis)
glossospasm (glos′ ō spa zm)
hepatitis (hep a tī′ tis)
hepatomegaly (hep a tō meg′ a lē)
hepatorrhagia (hep a tō rä′ jē a)
hypoglossal (hī′ pō glos′ əl)
pancreatectomy
    (pan krē a tek′ tō mē)
proctoclysis (prok tok′ li sis)
proctoscopy (prok tos′ kō pē)
rectal (rek′ t'l)
stomatitis (stō mä tī′ tis)
stomatorrhagia (stō mät ō rä′ jē ə)

Unit 5 Self-Test

Part 1

From the list on the right, select the correct meaning for each of the following often used medical terms.

_____ 1. Proctoclysis

_____ 2. Stomatoplasty

_____ 3. Hepatectomy

_____ 4. Stomatorrhagia

_____ 5. Colic

_____ 6. Enteroclysis

_____ 7. Glossospasm

_____ 8. Dental

_____ 9. Enterotoxin

_____ 10. Cheilitis

_____ 11. Colostomy

_____ 12. Gastrectasia

_____ 13. Cheiloplasty

_____ 14. Hepatomegaly

_____ 15. Proctoscopy

a. Make a new opening in the colon

b. Abnormal enlargement of the liver

c. Of or pertaining to teeth

d. Intestinal poisoning

e. Stretching, dilation of the stomach

f. Spasm of the tongue

g. Hemorrhage of the mouth

h. Irrigation of the rectum and anus

i. Plastic surgery of the mouth

j. Relating to the colon

k. Plastic surgery of the lips

l. Irrigation of the intestine

m. Surgical removal of (part of) the liver

n. Examination (looking into) the rectum through the anus with an endoscope

o. Inflammation of the lips

Part 2

Complete each of the medical terms on the right with the appropriate terms.

1. Under the tongue _____

2. Surgical removal of the pancreas _____

3. Hemorrage of the mouth _____

4. Inflammation of the lips _____

5. Enlarged liver _____

6. Stretching or dilation of the stomach _____

7. Spasm of the tongue _____

8. Plastic surgery of the lips _____

9. Intestinal hernia _____

10. Inflammation of the liver _____

11. Instrument for examining the rectum
    and anus _____

12. Pertaining to the rectum _____

13. Formation of a new opening in the
    colon _____

14. Painful tongue _____

15. Irrigation of the rectum and anus _____

ANSWERS

Part 1	*Part 2*
1. h	1. Hypoglossal
2. i	2. Pancreatectomy
3. m	3. Stomatorrhagia
4. g	4. Cheilitis
5. j	5. Hepatomegaly
6. l	6. Gastrectasia
7. f	7. Glossospasm
8. c	8. Cheiloplasty
9. d	9. Enterocele
10. o	10. Hepatitis

11. a	11. Proctoscope
12. e	12. Rectal
13. k	13. Colostomy
14. b	14. Glossalgia
15. n	15. Proctoclysis

6 The Heart

Unit 6 focuses on the gross anatomy of the heart and how the heart works. You'll create terms relating to abnormal conditions of the heart, and its abnormal functions. You'll also cover some new prefixes and suffixes as shown below.

Mini-Glossary

algesia (sense of pain)

angi/o (vessel)

arteri/o (artery)

cardiac arrest (stopped heart)

dactyl/o (fingers)

defibrillation (heart shocked to a regular heartbeat)

embolism (obstruction of a blood vessel)

embolus (foreign particle in the bloodstream)

esthesia (feeling, sensation)

fibrillation (very fast, irregular heartbeat)

myel/o (spinal cord, bone marrow)

phas/o (speech)

phleb/o (vein)

plas/o (formation)

thrombosis (bloodclot occluding a vessel)

thrombus (a blood clot)

a-, an- (absent, without)

dys- (bad, difficult, painful)

-emia (blood)

macro- (large)

micro- (small, very small)

poly- (many)

sym-, syn- (together)

-orrhexis (rupture, bursting apart)

-tripsy (rubbing, crushing)

Before you begin Unit 6, take the time to complete the Review Sheet for Unit 5. It will refresh your memory of the terms and word parts you studied. Find out how much you've learned.

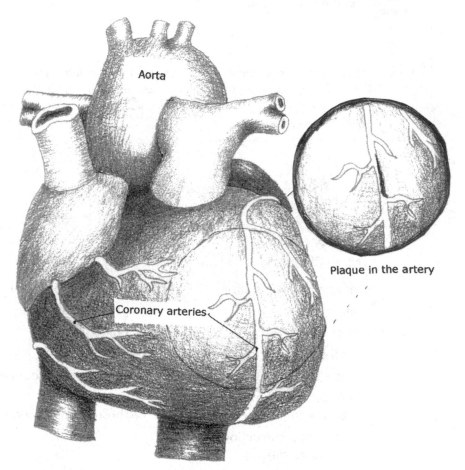

Aorta

Plaque in the artery

Coronary arteries

Figure 6.1. Coronary Arteries—Nourishment to the Heart

The *heart* is the pump of the circulatory system. It is about the size of a fist. It's hollow and cone-shaped, with its apex at the bottom. The heart uses arteries to deliver oxygen-rich blood to the cells, tissues, and organs. Oxygen-depleted blood returns to the heart via the veins. The heart then pumps oxygen-deficient blood to the lungs where it becomes oxygen-enriched and returns to the heart for another circulatory round.

The *coronary arteries* are so-named because they form an upside down "crown" on the surface of the heart. Both left and right arteries arise from small openings in the *aorta* just beyond the left side of the heart. The two main arteries form many branches and terminate in multitudes of tiny arteries that pass into the heart muscle and supply it with oxygen and nutrients.

Atherosclerotic plaque within the coronary artery may reduce blood flow and cause insufficient oxygen to reach the heart muscle. This condition often induces sharp, crushing chest pain. *Coronary thrombosis* means the coronary vessel may be occluded. Consequently, if the heart muscle is severely damaged, *fibrillation* may occur, and/or *cardiac arrest* may follow.

1.

Let's try something different. Some terms referring to abnormal conditions of the heart or blood vessels can be confusing. Read each definition carefully and select the terms that refer to a condition or procedure involving only the heart. Put an X in the box.

☐ (thrombus) ☐ *Thrombus* is a circulating blood clot.
☒ (coronary thrombosis) ☐ *Coronary thrombosis* is a heart attack caused by a blood clot that occludes (closes off) a coronary vessel of the heart.
☐ (embolus) ☐ *Embolus* is a foreign or abnormal particle circulating in the blood, such as a bubble of air, a blood clot, or cholesterol plaque.
☐ (embolism) ☐ *Embolism* is the sudden obstruction of a blood vessel by an embolus.
☒ cardiac arrest ☐ *Cardiac arrest* is the complete cessation of heart function. (If the heartbeat cannot be restored, the patient dies.)
☒ fibrillation ☐ *Fibrillation* means very fast and irregular heartbeat.
☒ defibrillation ☐ *Defibrillation* means using an electrical spark to shock the heart and bring about a slower and regular heartbeat.

Now review the terms and their meanings again. This time *circle* each term that refers to a condition of the blood or blood vessels.

2.

Try these. A blood clot floating through the blood stream is known as a *thrombus*. When a blood clot occludes a vessel, the condition is called *thrombosis*. The part of the word meaning abnormal or diseased condition is _____.

–osis

3.

Refer to the definitions in Frame 1. An embolus is any foreign or abnormal particle circulating in the blood, such as an air bubble, a cholesterol deposit, or even a blood clot. Embolism is the condition caused by an _____.

embolus
em′ bō lus

thrombus
throm′ bus
embolus

A circulating blood clot is a _____. But any foreign particle (including a blood clot) circulating through the bloodstream is an _____.

4.

embol (ism)   When a vessel is suddenly occluded by an embolus, the resulting
em′ bō lizm   condition is known as an _____ism.

thromb (osis) When a sudden vessel occlusion is caused by a thrombus, the result-
throm bō′ sis ing condition is a _____osis.

thrombosis   A blood clot occluding a coronary (heart) vessel is a condition
               called coronary _____.

5.

embolus   Embolism is caused by a/an _____.

thrombus   Thrombosis is caused by a/an _____.

6.

               A sudden blocking or occlusion of the coronary vessel of the heart by
coronary thrombosis a blood clot is a/an _____ _____.

7.

Cardiac fibrillation may result from coronary thrombosis. The heart
beats 200 to 400 times a minute and is very irregular. If something
is not done quickly, fibrillation will exhaust the heart and it will
stop beating altogether.

On the other hand, using an electrical spark to shock the heart
and bring about a slower and regular heartbeat may result in *de*fibrillation.

defibrillation   Underline the term that indicates the better outcome:
dē fib ri lā′ shun cardiac arrest / defibrillation

8.

               A very fast, irregular heartbeat, left unchecked, may lead to a com-
               plete cessation of heart functioning known as _____
cardiac arrest _____.

9.

               A very fast, irregular heartbeat is called fibrillation. Using an elec-
               trical spark to shock the heart and bring about a regular heartbeat is
defibrillation called _____.

10.

Write the correct term for each of the following definitions:

thrombus

a blood clot floating through the bloodstream, _____;

defibrillation

using an electrical spark to shock the heart and restore a regular heartbeat, _____;

cardiac arrest

complete cessation of heart functioning, _____ _____;

fibrillation

a very fast, irregular heartbeat, _____;

embolism

sudden blocking or occlusion of a vessel by something that floated in the bloodstream, _____;

coronary thrombosis

sudden blocking of the coronary vessel by a blood clot, _____ _____.

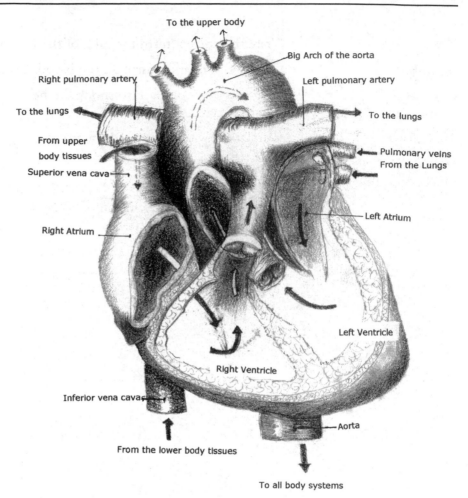

To the upper body

Big Arch of the aorta

Right pulmonary artery

Left pulmonary artery

To the lungs

To the lungs

From upper body tissues

Pulmonary veins From the Lungs

Superior vena cava

Left Atrium

Right Atrium

Left Ventricle

Right Ventricle

Inferior vena cava

Aorta

From the lower body tissues

To all body systems

Figure 6.2   The Cardiovascular System

The *heart* is the muscular pump of the cardiovascular system. It pumps blood to the lungs and body systems and receives blood back for recirculation. Each day, the heart beats about 100,000 times at a rate of approximately 70 beats per minute.

The heart contains four cavities, or chambers: two on the right side (pulmonary heart), two on the left (systemic heart). Pulmonary circulation carries blood to and from the lungs. The systemic circulation supplies oxygen- and nutrient-rich blood to the body cells, tissues, and organs. After completing the systemic circuit, all blood returns to the heart through the two main veins, the *superior vena cava* and the *inferior vena cava*.

These vena cavae meet at the *right atrium*, a thin-walled chamber that serves as a collecting station. From the right atrium, the blood flows downward into the *right ventricle*, the smaller of the two muscular heart chambers. When the ventricle contracts, blood is forced upward, as in the illustration. It is pumped through the *right and left pulmonary arteries*, which lead to the two lungs. This begins the pulmonary circuit. Blood is pumped to the lungs for oxygenation then returns to the heart for distribution to the body.

Blood from the lungs returns to the *left atrium* of the heart via the *pulmonary veins*. The veins are shown only on the left side of the heart; in the illustration they are hidden on the right side. From the left atrium (a collecting station) blood flows downward and enters the *left ventricle*, which is the larger of the two side-by-side muscular chambers. When the ventricles contract, simultaneously, the oxygenated blood is forced upward from the left ventricle through the big arch and into the aorta. Arteries arising from the aorta reach all parts of the head, upper extremities, thorax, abdomen, pelvic cavity, and lower extremities. The blood nourishes the tissues and returns to the heart to complete the circulation.

artery (arteri/o)	vein (phleb/o)
vessel (angi/o)	lung (pneumon/o)

11.
Arteries are vessels that carry blood *away* from the heart. Veins are vessels that carry blood *back to* the _____.

heart

12.
Note: Angi/o is the term used for vessels, whether the vessel is an artery or a vein.

What is a cardioangiogram? _____
_____.

a radiographic picture
    of the heart vessels
    (arteries and veins)

13.
A combining form for vein is phleb/o. If arteriosclerosis is hardening of the _____,

then hardening of veins is called

_____ / _____ / _____ / _____.
      vein   hardening   condition

arteries
phleb/o/scler/osis
phlebosclerosis
flēb′ ō skler ō′ sis

14.
Build a word meaning incision into a vein (venisection or cut down), _____ / _____;

inflammation of a vein, _____ / _____.

phleb/otomy
phlebotomy
flē bot′ ō mē

phleb/itis
phlebitis
flē bī′ tis

clot

15.
Thromb/o is the combining form that means clot.
Thromb/o/angi/itis means inflammation of a vessel with formation
of a _____.

excision of a thrombus
(clot)

16.
Thromb/ectomy means _____
_____.

inflammation of a vein
with thrombus
formation

17.
Thromb/o/phleb/itis means _____
_____
_____.

thrombus

18.
A synonym for clot is _____.

thromb/osis
thrombosis
throm bō′ sis

19.
Build a word meaning a condition caused by a clot,
_____ / _____;

thromb/o/cyte
thrombocyte
throm′ bō sīt

a cell that aids in clotting,
_____ / _____ / _____;

thromb/oid
thromboid
throm′ boid

resembling a clot,
_____ / _____.

20.
Let's review. Add the correct term to each of the definitions below.

Cardiac arrest

_____ _____ is the complete cessation
of heart function.

Coronary thrombosis

_____ is a heart attack caused by a blood clot
occluding the coronary blood vessel.

Defibrillation

_____ is a procedure using an electrical spark to
shock the heart and bring about a regular heartbeat.

Embolism

_____ is the sudden obstruction of a blood vessel
by an embolus.

Embolus

_____ is a foreign or abnormal particle circulating
in the bloodstream such as an air bubble, fat globule, or cholesterol
plaque.

Fibrillation   _____ means a very fast (200–400 beats/min) and irregular heartbeat.

Thrombus   _____ is a blood clot in the blood stream.

In this next section, you are taking on some new suffixes and pre-fixes.

21.
From the suggested answers select the meaning of each of the combining forms listed below.

SUGGESTED ANSWERS
blood vessel   blood clot
artery   vein
lung(s)

arteri/o _____
thromb/o _____
phleb/o _____
angi/o _____
pulmon/o _____

It's time to take a short break.

22.
Try this one.

-Orrhexis is a suffix meaning rupture.

Cyst/orrhexis means _____

rupture of the bladder   _____.

rupture of the small intestine   Enter/orrhexis means _____
_____.

rupture of a blood vessel   Angi/orrhexis means _____
_____.

cardi/orrhexis
cardiorrhexis
kär dē ō rek′ sis

23.
Build a word meaning rupture of the heart,
_____ / _____;

phleb/orrhexis
phleborrhexis
flē bŏ rek′ sis

rupture of a vein,
_____ / _____.

24.

Here's a chance to use all the "orrh" suffixes with some combining forms to help you.

-orrhexis means rupture, bursting apart
-orrhagia means burst forth, hemorrhage
-orrhaphy means repair, suture together, close
-orrhea means flow, discharge

rhin/o   saliping/o
cyst/o   hepat/o

Build a medical term to satisfy each of the following definitions.

rupture of the (urinary) bladder

cyst/orrhexis

_____ / _____ ;

hemorrhage from the liver,

hepat/orrhagia

_____ / _____ ;

flowing from the nose (runny nose),

rhin/orrhea

_____ / _____ ;

suturing (or joining) the fallopian tubes,

salping/orrhaphy

_____ / _____ .

suturing (or closing) a
   rupture, hernia

What does herniorrhaphy mean? _____

_____ .

25.
Fill in the blank to complete these definitions

SUGGESTED ANSWERS
-orrhagia   -orrhaphy
-orrhea   -orrhexis

-orrhaphy   _____ means repair, close, suture
-orrhagia   _____ means burst forth, hemorrhage
-orrhea   _____ means discharge, flowing
-orrhexis   _____ means rupture, bursting apart

26.
An- is a form of the prefix *a-* meaning without. *Esthesia* means feeling or sensation. Give the meaning of the following words:

anesthesia _____

a condition of being   _____
   without feeling   _____ ;

the study or science of
removing feeling

anesthesiology _____

_____

_____ ;

instrument for
measuring feeling or
sensation

esthesiometer _____

_____

_____ ;

abnormal sensitivity
(to pain)

hyperesthesia _____

_____ .

27.

Analyze the following words (you do the dividing):

an/esthesi/o/log/ist
an′ es thēz ē ol′ ō jist

anesthesiologist, _____ ;

hypo/esthes/ia
hī pō es thē′ zē ə

hypoesthesia, _____ .

28.

Algesia is a word meaning a sense of pain. What does analgesia
mean? _____

without sensitivity to
pain
an′ al jē′ zē ə

_____ .

29.

The prefixes *a-* and *an-* mean without. Examine the following two
lists of words:

an/*algesia*   a/*biotic*
an/*emia*   a/*dermia*
an/*encephalus*   a/*febrile*
an/*esthesia*   a/*kinesia*
an/*onychia*   a/*menia*
an/*opia*   a/*menorrhea*
an/*uria*   a/*pnea*
an/*uresis*   a/*sepsis*

Draw a conclusion: When the word root begins with a consonant,
use the prefix _____ .

a-

an-

When the word root begins with a vowel, use the prefix _____ .

30.

Put the proper form of the prefix before each of the following roots
and then write a meaning for each.

*an*emic—a condition of
less blood

_____emic _____

_____ ;

*a*stomia—without a
mouth (congenital)

_____stomia _____

_____;

*a*febrile—without fever   _____febrile _____;

*an*odontia— toothless   _____odontia _____.

31.
Here's some practice with other prefixes. *Phas/o* means speech.
Write a meaning for each of the following:

speechless   aphasia _____;

tachyphasia _____

abnormally fast speech   _____;

bradyphasia _____

abnormally slow speech   _____;

pain or difficulty when   dysphasia _____
speaking

_____.

32.
pain along the course   *Neur/o* is used in words that refer to nerves. Neur/algia means
of a nerve (or
equivalent)   _____

_____.

33.
Tripsis, from which we get trips/y, is a Greek word that means
"rub" or "massage." Neur/o/trips/y means surgical crushing of a
nerve. The word root for crushing (usually by rubbing or grinding)
trips   is _____.

neur/o/trips/y   Tripsis can be carried to the point of crushing or grinding. Surgical
neurotripsy   crushing of a nerve is called
nyoo' rō trip sē   _____ / _____ / _____ / _____.

34.
In some cases of cholelithiasis, it may be necessary to crush calculi
chole/lith/o/trips/y   so they can pass from the gallbladder. A word meaning surgical
cholelithotripsy   crushing of gallstones is
kō lē lith' ō trip sē   _____ / _____ / _____ / _____ / _____.

35.
Myel/itis can mean either inflammation of bone marrow or inflammation of the spinal cord. From the definitions, you may conclude

bone marrow spinal cord	that *myel* can be the word root for both _____ and _____.
	36. The suffix -*blast* means an immature cell (in the process of developing). In the term myel/o/blast, the word root myel refers to bone marrow. Write the meaning of myel/o/blast: _____
an immature bone marrow cell	_____.
hernia of the spinal cord	In myel/o/cele, the word root refers to spinal cord. Write the meaning of myel/o/cele: _____ _____.
bone marrow or spinal cord	**37.** A medical term built on the word root myel may refer to different structures of the body. It may refer to either _____ or _____
	38. You have learned that dys- means pain, painful. But dys- is a prefix that also means bad (defective) or difficult. Try this. *Plasia* means formation or change, in the sense of molding during the *growing years*. This kind of formation occurs naturally instead of being done by a plastic surgeon. Dys/plasia means _____
bad, defective (poor or abnormal formation)	_____.
hyper/plasia hyperplasia hī′ per plā′ zha	**39.** A/plasia means failure of an organ to develop properly. A term that means overgrowth or excessive development in the formative years is _____ / _____.
hypo/plasia hypoplasia hī′ pō plā′ zha	**40.** If overdevelopment is hyperplasia, underdevelopment is expressed as _____ / _____.
chondr/o/dys/plasia chondrodysplasia kon′ drō dis plā′ zhə bad (defective) development of cartilage	**41.** Myel/o/dys/plasia means defective development of the spinal cord. What does chondr/o/dys/plasia mean? _____ _____.

oste/o/chondr/o/dys/
  plasia
osteochondrodysplasia
os′ tē ō kon′ drō dis
  plā′ zhə
defective formation of
  bone and cartilage

42.
Write the meaning of osteochondrodysplasia. _____

_____

_____.

43.
Here's another quick review before moving on.

SUGGESTED ANSWERS
-algesia   phas/o
-dys   plas/o
-tripsy   lith/o
               myel/o

Write the suffix or combining form that refers to each of the following words.

myel/o
phas/o
-algesia
lith/o
-tripsy
myel/o
dys-
plas/o

spinal cord _____
speech _____
sensation of pain _____
calculus _____
rubbing, crushing (procedure) _____
bone marrow _____
painful, difficult, bad _____
formation, development _____

44.
Explain the meaning of the following medical terms.

abnormally slow speech
rubbing, crushing of a
  nerve
incision to remove a
  gallstone
radiographic exam of
  the spinal cord
bad development
  (formation) of
  cartilage
lack of pain sensation

bradyphasia _____
neurotripsy _____
_____
cholelithotomy _____
_____
myelogram _____
_____
chondrodysplasia _____
_____
_____
analgesia _____
_____

45.

microns
mī′ krons

micr/o/meter
micrometer
mī krom′ ə ter

The *micron* (1/1000 mm) is a unit of measurement. Many cocci are 2 microns in diameter. A red blood cell is 7 _____ in diameter.

An instrument for measuring the diameter of something microscopic is a _____ / _____ / meter.

46.

large

On the other hand, *macr/o* is the opposite of micr/o. Macr/o is used in words to mean _____.

47.

a large immature cell
    visible by the naked
    eye

Things that are macr/o/scop/ic can be seen with the naked eye. Give a meaning for macroblast. _____

_____

_____.

48.

Macr/o/cephal/us
mak rō se fal′ us

An abnormally large head is

_____ / _____ / _____ / _____.

macr/o/cyte

An abnormally large cell is a

_____ / _____ / _____.

macr/o/cocc/us

A very large coccus is called a

_____ / _____ / _____ / _____.

49.

In each case there is a
    condition of—

abnormally large tongue
mak rō glos′ ē ə
abnormally large ear(s)
mak rō′ shē ə
abnormally large nose
mak rō rin′ ē ə
abnormally large lips
mak rō kē′ lē ə

The suffix -ia indicates a condition. Pronounce each term and write a meaning.

Macr/o/gloss/ia _____

_____

Macr/ot/ia _____

_____

Macr/o/rhin/ia _____

_____

Macr/o/cheil/ia _____

_____

50.

dactyl
dak′ til

Macr/o/dactyl/ia means abnormally large fingers or toes. The word root for fingers or toes is _____.

englarged digits, or another way of saying large fingers or toes

51.
What does dactyl/o/megaly mean? _____.

52.
A finger or toe is called a digit or dactyl. But the combining form

dactyl/o

for digit is _____ / _____.

dactyl/itis
dactylitis
dak til ī′ tis

Build a term meaning inflammation of a digit,

_____ / _____;

dactyl/o/spasm
dactylospasm
dak til′ ō spa zm

cramp or spasm of a digit,

_____ / _____ / _____;

dactyl/o/gram
dactylogram
dak til′ ō gram

a fingerprint,

_____ / _____ / _____.

abnormally large fingers and toes (digits)

53.
Macr/o/dactyl/ia means _____

_____.

fingers or toes (digits)

Poly/dactyl/ism means too many _____

_____.

poly/ur/ia
polyuria
pol ē yer′ ē ə

54.
Poly- is a prefix meaning too many or too much. Poly/ur/ia means excessive amount of urine. When a person drinks a lot of fluid,

_____ / _____ / _____ results.

polyneuritis
pol ē nyo͞o rī′ tis

55.
Path refers to disease.

Poly/neur/o/path/y means disease of many nerves.

inflammation of many nerves

What does poly/neur/itis mean? _____

_____.

inflammation of many joints

56.
Write the meaning of the following:
Poly/arthr/itis _____

_____;

pain in several nerves

Poly/neur/algia _____

_____.

syn/ergetic synergetic sin er je' tik	**57.** Syn/ergetic means working together. Drugs that work together to increase the effects of one another are called _____ / _____ drugs.
synergetic	**58.** Synergetic muscles are muscles that work together. Three muscles work together to flex the forearm. The function of these muscles is described as _____.
synergetic	**59.** APC tablets are thought by some to be more effective for killing pain than aspirin alone. This is because *a*spirin, *p*henacetin, and *c*affeine are _____ drugs.
a fused joint that moves as one	**60.** Syn/arthr/osis means an immovable joint; adjoining bones are fused together. When bones of a joint are fused so they all move as one, the condition is syn/arthr/osis. What does it mean? _____ _____.
<u>syn</u>dactylism <u>syn</u>arthrosis	Underline the part of the word that means joined together as one: syndactylism synarthrosis
a condition of two or more digits joined together as one	**61.** What does syn/dactyl/ism mean (–ism denotes a medical condition or disease)? _____ _____.
together or joined as one	**62.** *Syn-* and *sym-* are different forms of the same prefix: Syn- and sym- mean _____.
	63. Use the prefix sym- when the word root begins with the consonants b, m, or p; use syn- in all other cases. Write the prefix for each of the following:
<u>syn</u>arthrosis <u>sym</u>metrical <u>sym</u>bolism <u>sym</u>physis	_____ arthrosis _____ metrical _____ bolism _____ physis

syndrome   _____ drome
sympathy   _____ pathy
symbiosis   _____ biosis

64.
joined as one, together
b, m, p

Both syn- and sym- mean _____ _____; sym- is used when followed by the letters _____, _____, or _____; syn- is used in other medical words.

65.
Time to review. Complete each brief definition. Refer to the suggested answers. Write your selection in the space provided.

SUGGESTED ANSWERS:

algesia	phas/o
dactyl/o	phleb/o
embolus	plas/o
esthesia	

algesia
phleb/o
embolus
esthesia
phas/o
plas/o
dactyl/o

a sensation of pain _____
veins _____
foreign particle circulating in the blood _____
feeling, sensation _____
speech _____
formation, development _____
digits _____

66.
Try these.

SUGGESTED ANSWERS:

a-, an-	-orrhagia
dys-	-orrhaphy
macro-	-orrhexis
micro-	syn-, sym-
-orrhea	-tripsy

-orrhexis
syn-, sym-
dys-
-orrhagia
macro-
-tripsy

rupture, burst apart _____
together, as one _____
defective, difficult, painful _____
hemorrhage, burst forth _____
large _____
crushing, rubbing _____

micro–	microscopic, very small _____
-orrhea	flowing, discharge _____
a–, an–	without, absent _____
-orrhaphy	suturing (repair of) _____

67.

In your own words, write the meaning for each of the following:

Here are some suggestions:

neur/o/tripsy

crushing of a nerve
_____

without sensation of pain

an/esthesia
_____

bad formation of the spinal cord

myel/o/dys/plasia
_____

a condition of a blood clot in the coronary artery

coronary thrombosis
_____
_____

pertaining to something too small to see with the naked eye

micro/scop/ic
_____
_____

without speech, speechless

a/phasia
_____

a condition of fingers joined together as one

syn/dactyl/ism
_____

surgical repair of a hernia

herni/orrhaphy
_____

hepat/orrhagia

hemorrhage of the liver
_____

an/algesia

without, or absent, pain
_____

complete cessation of heart function

cardiac arrest
_____

electrical shock of the heart to restore regular rhythm

defibrillation
_____
_____

ruptured blood vessel (vein)

phleb/orrhexis
_____

68.

Here are 30 medical terms for practicing your pronunciation. Say the term aloud and then say what it means. Then take the Unit 6 Self-Test.

analgesia (an′ al jē′ zē ə)

anemia (an ē′ mē ə)

anesthesiologist
   (an′ es thē zē ol′ ō jist)

angiogram (an′ gē ō gram)

cardiorrhexis (kär dē ōr rek′ sis)

chondrodysplasia
   (kon′ drō dis plā′ zhə)

cystorrhexis (sis tō rek′ sis)

dactylogram (dak til′ ō gram)

dactylomegaly
   (dak′ til ō meg′ ə lē)

defibrillation (dē fib ri lā′ shun)

embolism (em′bō lizm)

embolus (em′ bō lus)

esthesiometer
   (es thē zē om′ ə ter)

hyperesthesia
   (hī′ per es thē′ zhə)

hypoesthesia (hī′ pō es thē′ zhə)

hypoplasia (hī′ pō plā′ zhə)

hysterorrhexis (his′ ter ō rek′ sis)

lithotripsy (lith′ ō trip sē)

macrocephalus
   (mak′ rō se fal′ us)

macrocheilia (mak′ rō kē′ lē ə)

macrotia (mak rō′ shē ə)

micrometer (mī krom′ ə ter)

neuromyelitis
   (nyoo′ rō mī il ī′ tis)

neurotripsy (nyoo′ rō trip sē)

phlebitis (flē bī′ tis)

polyarthritis (pol ē arth rī′ tis)

polyuria (pol ē yer′ ē ə)

syndactylism (sin dak′ til izm)

thrombosis (throm bō′ sis)

thrombus (throm′ bus)

Unit 6 Self-Test

Part 1

From the list on the right, select the correct meaning for each of the following often used medical terms. Put the letter in the space provided.

_____ 1. Lithotripsy

_____ 2. Thrombosis

_____ 3. Polyarthritis

_____ 4. Anesthetist

_____ 5. Synarthrosis

_____ 6. Phlebitis

_____ 7. Hysterorrhexis

_____ 8. Dactylogram

_____ 9. Analgesia

_____ 10. Defibrillation

_____ 11. Neuromyelitis

_____ 12. Macrocephalus

_____ 13. Hypoesthesia

_____ 14. Embolism

_____ 15. Aphasia

a. Inflammation of a vein

b. Shocking the heart to restore a normal heartbeat

d. Obstruction of a blood vessel by an embolus

e. Abnormally enlarged head

f. Absence of pain

g. Inflammation of many joints

i. A specialist who removes all feeling or sensation

j. Crushing of a calculus

k. Bursting apart of the uterus

l. Fingerprint

m. Speechless

n. Clotted condition of a blood vessel

o. Inflammation of the nerves of the spinal cord

p. Less than normal sensation

q. Immovable joint, bones of a joint joined together as one

Part 2

Complete each of the medical terms on the right with the appropriate missing part or word.

1. Rupture (bursting apart) of the urinary bladder _____

2. Abnormally intense feeling or sensation _____

3. Foreign particle occluding a blood vessel _____ism

4. Rupture (bursting apart) of the heart _____

5. Abnormally large head _____

6. Inflammation of many nerves _____

7. Pain along the course of a nerve _____

8. A stopped heart _____(2 wds)

9. Abnormally large fingers _____

10. Foreign substance circulating in the bloodstream _____

11. Instrument for measuring feeling, sensation _____

12. A blood clot circulating in the bloodstream _____

13. Crushing destruction of a nerve _____

14. Absent the ability to speak, speechless _____

15. Fingers grown together as one _____

ANSWERS

Part 1	*Part 2*
1. j.	1. Cystorrhexis
2. n.	2. Hyperesthesia
3. g.	3. Embolism
4. i.	4. Cardiorrhexis
5. q.	5. Macrocephalus
6. a.	6. Polyneuritis
7. k.	7. Neuralgia
8. l.	8. Cardiac arrest

9. f.	9.	Dactylomegaly
10. b.	10.	Embolus
11. o.	11.	Esthesiometer
12. e.	12.	Thrombus
13. p.	13.	Neurotripsy
14. d.	14.	Aphasia
15. m.	15.	Syndactylism

7 Symptoms, Diagnoses, Treatments, Communication Qualifiers, and Statistics

In this unit you will learn many terms related to signs and symptoms, diagnoses, treatments, and statistics. Some words will be familiar, but you'll use them in new ways.

Signs

atrophy
edema
hypertrophy
pulse
respiration
temperature

Qualifiers

acute
central
chronic
generalized
localized
paroxysmal
peripheral

Word Parts

anti- (*against*)
chlor/o (*green*)
erythr/o (*red*)
melan/o (*black*)
pyret/o (*fever*)
xanth/o (*yellow*)

Symptoms

anorexia
dyspnea
malaise
nausea
tinnitus
vertigo

Treatments

active
palliative
prophylactic
systemic

Diagnosis

prodrome
prognosis
syndrome

Statistics

morbidity
mortality

Be sure to complete the Unit 6 Review Sheet before continuing.

Signs and Symptoms

1.

What is a sign or a symptom? Let's take them one at a time. A *sign* is any abnormality of the body a physician may discover on examination of the patient. A *symptom* is also evidence of an abnormality in structure or function. However, the patient experiences a symptom through one or more of the five organs of sense. Can you name them?

sight
sound
smell
taste
feel

_____   _____   _____   _____   _____

2.

Simply put, a sign or a symptom is evidence there is something wrong. The patient feels, tastes, or hears something that is out of the ordinary and tells the examiner about it. This symptomatic evidence may not be apparent to the examiner. On the other hand, sometimes evidence can be observed by the examiner and also be experienced by the patient. Check the box that indicates whether the evidence described is a sign, a symptom, or both.

	SIGN	SYMPTOM	BOTH	
both	☐	☐	☐	swelling of the wrist
symptom	☐	☐	☐	ringing (tinkling sound) in the ear
symptom	☐	☐	☐	sourness in the mouth
symptom	☐	☐	☐	ammonia sensation in the nose
both	☐	☐	☐	painful and swollen elbow
both	☐	☐	☐	bleeding from the nose
both	☐	☐	☐	blue discoloration around the eye
both	☐	☐	☐	very rapid breathing
symptom	☐	☐	☐	pain in the heel
both	☐	☐	☐	chills and fever
both	☐	☐	☐	painful muscle spasm in the leg
both	☐	☐	☐	chills, coughing, and runny nose
sign	☐	☐	☐	slow heartbeat
sign	☐	☐	☐	pale complexion
sign	☐	☐	☐	eyes closed, not responding to questions or poking

3.

An abnormality apparent to an examiner (and sometimes to the patient) is called a _____.

sign

4.

symptom

Any change in body function or structure that the patient sees, hears, tastes, smells, or feels (and may not be apparent to an observer) is called a _____.

As you can see, most evidence of illness can be observed by someone other than the patient and may be experienced by the patient as well.

Vital Signs

5.

vital signs

Vital means relating to life. A vital sign is evidence a patient is alive. Body temperature, pulse rate, and rate of respiration are vital signs because they provide continuous information about the essential processes of the body. If one of these signs is absent, the patient is dead (or in big trouble). Body temperature, pulse, and respiration are very important indicators and are called _____.

6.

98.6

Vital signs can be measured. Temperature (T) loosely refers to body heat above normal. Normal body temperature is 98.6°F. Body temperature increases in a hot environment and during physical exercise. Many diseases, serious and not serious, cause a patient's temperature to rise. Elevated body temperature is called *fever.* Low fever is 99° to 101°F. Moderate fever is 101° to 103°F. High fever is 103° to 105°F. A patient who is afebrile has a normal body temperature, which is approximately _____ °F.

7.

fires

Pyro is a word root meaning fire or heat. (Remember the funeral pyres on which the Greeks and Romans burned their dead?) A pyromaniac has a fondness for watching things burn or starting _____.

8.

above

Pyret/o forms words meaning fever. A patient described as pyretic would have a temperature _____98.6°F.

(above/below/same as)

9.

sign

Pyrexia means feverish. Fever is one way the body shows something is wrong. Fever can be observed and measured; therefore, pyrexia is a _____ of disease.

sign/symptom

hypothermia
hī pō ther′ mē ə

10.
Hypo/thermia refers to body temperature below normal. A patient's temperature may be lowered safely to about 80° during surgery. This controlled procedure reduces the patient's need for oxygen and makes some surgical procedures safer. The patient's lower body temperature is called _____.

hypothermia

11.
On the other hand, a person who falls through the ice on a pond in January will surely develop a life-threatening condition also called _____.

hyper
hī per

12.
Injury and dehydration can cause a patient's temperature to rise above 106°F. This life-threatening high temperature is known as _____pyrexia.
(hyper/hypo)

that which produces
fever

13.
In an earlier unit you learned that gen/o means to produce or originate. What does pyret/o/gen mean? _____
_____.

pyretogen
pī ret′ō jen

14.
The measles virus produces fever. Therefore, the virus that causes measles is a _____.

pertains to something
that produces fever

15.
Pyret/ic means pertaining to fever. What does pyret/o/gen/ic mean? _____
_____.

an agent that works
against fever

16.
Anti- means against. Aspirin is an anti/pyret/ic agent. What does antipyretic mean? _____
_____.

fever reduction

17.
Lysis means dissolution or reduction. What does pyret/o/lysis mean? _____.

without symptoms

18.
A physician writes on a patient's chart, "The patient has a low-grade fever but is otherwise asymptomatic." What does asymptomatic mean? _____.

increase

19.
Now let's talk about another vital sign. Pulse (P) is a rhythmical throbbing of the arterial walls. This throbbing is produced when the heart contracts and forces an increased volume of blood into the vessels. After chasing your dog down the street, you would expect your pulse rate to _____.
(increase/decrease)

tachycardia

20.
The normal pulse of an average adult is 70 to 80 beats per minute. Fever usually causes a patient's heart to beat more rapidly. When a patient's pulse is 100 beats per minute or higher the condition is known as _____.
(tachycardia/bradycardia)

bradycardia

On the other hand, a pulse less than 60 beats per minute indicates _____.

sign

21.
The patient usually does not feel a rapid, slow, or irregular pulse. However, a physician can observe and measure pulse rate; therefore, it is said to be a _____.
(sign/symptom)

70 to 80

22.
Pulse rate depends on size, sex, age, and physical condition. It's higher in women than men. It's higher in children than adults. But we can say that a healthy adult has an average pulse of (Check one.)

☐   30 to 50 beats per minute.
☐   70 to 80 beats per minute.

vital sign

23.
The pulse is usually felt over the radial artery at the wrist. Although pulse is a simple measure, it provides important evidence about the life (and death) status of the patient. Therefore, it is considered a _____.

peripheral
per i′ fer al

24.
Periphery means outer surface of the body. It is the part of the body away from the center. A pulse taken at the wrist or ankle is a _____ pulse.
(central/peripheral)

central

25.
A pulse taken near the center of the body, where the heart is, is a _____ pulse.
(central/peripheral)

because it is near the
center of the body

26.
A pulse taken with a stethoscope on the chest is a central pulse. Why? _____
_____.

near the outer surface
of the body

27.
What does peripheral mean? _____
_____.

accelerated

28.
Here's the third vital sign. Respiration (R) is breathing. Breathing is a function of the respiratory system. A breath draws in oxygen. The circulating blood carries the oxygen to the tissues and then returns carbon dioxide to the lungs. The lungs breathe out the waste products of carbon dioxide and water. The normal rate of respiration for an adult is 16 to 18 breaths per minute. A respiration rate of more than 25 breaths per minute is _____ respiration.
(accelerated/decelerated)

an instrument for
measuring breathing

29.
Pne/o (pronounced nē o) means breath or breathing. Pne/o/dynamics means the mechanism of breathing. What does pne/o/meter mean? _____
_____.

30.
Here's a rule that will help you pronounce words containing the root pne/o, pne/a. When pne/o begins the word, the letter "p" is silent. The letter "p" is pronounced when a prefix comes before it. Pronounce each of the following:

a/pnea   pronounce: ap′ nē ə
hyper/pnea   pronounce: hī perp′ nē ə

tachy/pnea   pronounce: tak ip nē′ ə
brady/pnea   pronounce: brad′ ip nē ə
pneumon/ia   pronounce: nū mon′ ē ə

31.
Bradycardia means very slow heartbeat. What does brady/pnea mean? _____.

very slow breathing

32.
Pronounce dys/pnea. What does it mean? _____ _____.

disp′ nē ə
painful (bad) breathing

33.
Hyperpyrexia means excessively high temperature (over 106°F). What does hyperpnea mean? _____ _____.

excessively rapid
   breathing
hī perp′ nē ə

34.
A/symptomatic means without symptoms. What does a/pnea mean? _____.

without breathing

(Pronounce it.)

ap′ nē ə

35.
Fever and disorders of the lungs or heart may accelerate respiration. Build a word that describes a respiration rate over 25 breaths per minute: _____.

hyperpnea
hī perp′ nē ə

36.
Very slow breathing of 8 to 9 breaths per minute occurs in serious illnesses like uremia, diabetic coma, and opium poisoning. Build a term that means very slow breathing: _____.

bradypnea
brad ip nē′ ə

37.
A foreboding irregular and unusual pattern of breathing is called Cheyne-Stokes respiration. (Pronounced *chain-stokes*. It's a condition named after two physicians who first described it more than 150 years ago.) Respiration gradually increases in rapidity and volume until the rate reaches a climax (perhaps 60 to 80 breaths per minute). Then breathing subsides and ceases entirely for up to one minute—when respirations begin again. This condition is due to disturbance of the respiratory center in the brain. It is often a forerunner of death—but may last several months, days, or even disappear.

apnea
ap′ nē ə

38.
Cheyne-Stokes respiration is cyclical. The phase of respiration, at 60 to 80 breaths per minute, is called hyperpnea. What term describes the period when all respiration ceases? _____.

39.
In certain very serious illnesses, an irregular and arrythmic type of breathing may occur, characterized by both hyperpneic and apneic phases, often followed by death. It is called C_____-

Cheyne-Stokes

S_____ respiration.

40.
Something is very wrong with the body when a patient's respiration rate exceeds 25 breaths per minute. Respiration rate (R), fever (T), and a rapid pulse (P) are measurable signs of disease. They indicate

vital signs

the status of the whole body and are called _____ _____

temperature
pulse
respiration

41.
The vital signs are T _____, P _____, and R _____.

42.
Let's review. Select the best meaning from column B for each brief definition in column A. Write your selection in the space provided.

COLUMN A	COLUMN B
bodily change a patient perceives	asymptomatic

symptom
see, hear, smell, taste,
   feel

	vital signs
_____	hyperpyrexia
sensory ways symptoms are perceived	hypothermia
_____	pyretogen
temperature, pulse, and respiration	pyrteolysis

vital signs
pyrexia
pī rek′ sē ə
hypothermia
hī pō ther′ mē ə
hyperpyrexia
hī per pī rek′ se ə
pyretogen
pī ret′ ō gen
pyretolysis
pī ret ō lī′ sis
asymptomatic
ā simp tō mat′ ik

_____ _____	pyrexia
elevated temperature, fever	see, hear,
_____	smell,
subnormal body temperature	taste, feel
_____	symptom
temperature over 106°F	
_____	
something that produces fever	
_____	
reduction, dissolution of fever	
_____	
lack of symptoms	
_____	

43.

Now try these.

pulse

peripheral

pne/o, pne/a
bradypnea
dyspnea
hyperpnea
respiration
apnea

Cheyne-Stokes
respiration

COLUMN A	COLUMN B
throbbing of an artery in time with the heartbeat _____	apnea
	bradypnea
pulse taken at the surface of the body	Cheyne-
_____	Stokes
two combining forms for breath, breathing	respiration
_____ or _____	dyspnea
very slow breathing _____	hyperpnea
difficult breathing _____	peripheral
excessively fast breathing _____	pne/o, pne/a
another word for breathing _____	pulse
respiratory arrest, not breathing_____	respiration
breathing that reaches a climax, then ceases before beginning again _____ - _____	

Color and Other Signs

44.

Color and changes in color of various parts of the body also tell the physician a lot about the patient's condition. Use the information here to build words involving color.

leuk/o	white
melan/o	black
erythr/o	red
cyan/o	blue
chlor/o	green
xanth/o	yellow

xanth/opsia
zan thop′ sē ə
chlor/opia
klor ō′ pē ə

45.

Cyan/opia means blue vision. Form a word meaning

yellow vision, _____/<u>opsia</u>.

green vision, _____/<u>opia</u>.

erythr/o/derma
e rith′ rō der′ mä
melan/o/derma
mel′ a nō der′ mä

46.

Cyan/o/derma means blue skin. Build a word meaning

red skin, _____ / _____ / _____.

black (discolored) skin, _____.
(You draw the lines.)

47.
Write a meaning for each of the following:

green (plant) cell   chlor/o/cyte, _____.
white (blood) cell   leuk/o/cyte, _____.
red (blood) cell   erythr/o/cyte, _____.

48.
-Blast means immature cell. Build a word meaning an immature cell
of the following colors:

melan/o/blast
mel′ a nō blast   immature black cell, _____ / _____ / _____.
                                                      black   immature cell
erythr/o/blast
e rith′ rō blast   immature red cell, _____ / _____ / _____.

49.
Melan/osis means a condition of black pigmentation. Carcinoma is
a malignant tumor.

a black–pigmented   What is a melanocarcinoma? _____
   malignant tumor   _____.

50.
Whenever a hairless mole on the skin turns black and grows larger,
melanocarcinoma   a physician should be consulted because there is danger of black
mel′ a nō kär si nō′ mä   mole cancer, or _____.

51.
green   Chlor/o means _____.
red   Erythr/o means _____.
yellow   Xanth/o means _____.
white   Leuk/o means _____.

Qualifiers

52.
In medical terminology we often use qualifiers. These are adjectives
or adverbs that when used with another word make the meaning of
that term more specific. Here are a few frequently used qualifiers.
Local means a small area or part of the body. *General* means involving the whole body or many different areas or parts of the body at
the same time.

local

53.
Anesthesia may be considered either local or general. Before
extracting a tooth, the dentist injects Novocain to prevent pain.
Novocain is a _____ anesthetic.

(local/general)

general

54.
On the other hand, laughing gas, which puts the patient to sleep, is
a _____ anesthetic.

(local/general)

55.
Label each of the following as local or general.
skin rash around the neck and ears,

local

_____.

measles macules from stem to stern,

general

_____.

acne all over the face,

local

_____.

second-degree scalding burn over the belly and upper thigh,

local (two places)

_____.

reddish purple spots over the trunk of the body and wherever
clothing covers the skin,

general

_____.

a small area or part of
   the body

56.
A localized condition means _____
_____.

involving the whole
   body or many areas
   at the same time

When a condition is generalized, it means _____
_____.

general

57.
Systemic means pertaining to all body systems, or the whole body
rather than one of its parts. It is another word for _____.

(local/general)

systemic
sis tem′ ik
or general

58.
An antihistamine tablet helps a patient breathe more easily by dry-
ing up mucous membranes inside the nose and sinuses. An antihistamine also dries up mucous membranes that line all body cavities.
We say it has a _____ effect.

Other Signs

Besides observing color and color changes, a physician inspects the patient carefully for signs and symptoms that will aid in learning about a patient's disease. Here are some observable changes in the body.

fluid

59.
Edema refers to fluid in the tissues. It is a condition in which body tissues accumulate excessive _____.

the whole body

60.
Fluid in the tissues may be local or general. Localized edema involves a small area of the body; generalized edema involves _____.

edema
e dē′ ma

61.
A bee sting produces an accumulation of fluid in the tissues at the bite site. This is called localized _____.

generalized edema

62.
Heart failure causes severe disturbance of the body's water balance mechanisms. Excessive fluid may accumulate in the lungs, legs, and abdomen. This condition is called _____
(two words).   (localized/generalized)

edema

63.
Excessive accumulation of fluid in the body tissues is called _____.

Atrophy
at′ rō fē

64.
Atrophy is another observable sign of disease. It means a wasting away or shrinking of tissues, an organ, or the whole body. Underline the word root meaning development.

Atrophy

What does hyper/troph/y mean?

overdevelopment

_____.

65.
It's time to review. Select the best meaning from Column B for each color listed in Column A Write your selection in the space provided.

	COLUMN A	COLUMN B
erythr/o	red _____	cyan/o
leuk/o	white _____	chlor/o
cyan/o	blue _____	erythr/o
chlor/o	green _____	melan/o
xanth/o	yellow _____	leuk/o
melan/o	black _____	xanth/o

66.
Select a suggested answer to complete each of the following definitions.

SUGGESTED ANSWERS

edema	local
generalized	systemic
hypertrophy	atrophy

generalized

a) _____ means pertaining to the whole body or many areas at the same time.

systemic

b) Another term meaning the same as a) above is _____.

c) An injection of anesthetic under the skin of the forearm to

local

remove a mole is described as a _____ anesthetic.

d) Accumulated excess fluid in the tissues of the lower extremities

edema

may be a condition of _____.

e) A wasting away or shrinking of tissues of an organ or a body part

atrophy

is described as _____.

hypertrophy

f) _____ is the term that describes the opposite of e) above.

Subjective Symptoms

Objective *signs* such as T, P, and R are *signs* of primary importance in the investigation of an illness. However, the patient's own concerns and impressions also provide valuable information. Changes in the body not apparent to an observer but experienced by the patient are called *symptoms*.

67.
Nausea means sickness of the stomach with a desire to vomit. Since it is an internal feeling evident only to the patient, we call it a

symptom

_____.

68.
nausea
naw′ zē ə

Pain, noxious odors, fevers, and some drugs may cause a sickness of the stomach with a desire to vomit, which is called _____.

69.
nausea

Mal de mer is the French term meaning motion sickness. It is another way to describe the sick feeling of _____.

70.
emesis (or vomitus)
em′ e sis

Emesis means vomitus—that which is vomited. An irritation of the vomiting center in the brain produces nausea. As a result, the patient ejects the stomach contents through the mouth. The product of vomiting is _____.

71.
vomiting
emesis

Food poisoning, drugs, and fevers can irritate the vomiting center and thus induce _____. The product of vomiting is _____.

72.
blood in the vomitus

Chol/emesis means bile in the vomitus. What does hemat/emesis mean? _____
_____.

73.
pertaining to something that induces vomiting

In an emergency, there are two quick ways to empty the stomach of its contents: (a) use a tube to "pump" the stomach, or (b) give the patient an emetic. What is an emetic? _____
_____.

74.
(nausea) the patient feels the sensation (not observable)

Nausea usually precedes *emesis.* Circle the term that is a subjective symptom. Why? _____
_____.

75.
malaise

In a wide variety of illnesses, two symptoms often occur together. We'll take them one at a time.

Malaise is a French word literally meaning ill at ease. Underline the part of the word meaning ill.

malaise
ma lā´z

76.
A patient with infectious mononucleosis may experience a vague sensation of not feeling well, or feeling ill at ease. The symptom is called _____.

the vague sensation of
 not feeling well

77.
Malaise is a symptom because the physician cannot observe malaise and does not experience the patient's sensation. Describe malaise.

_____

_____.

without an appetite
an o rek´ sē ə

78.
Orexia means appetite. What does an/orexia mean? _____

_____.

pertaining to something
 that produces or
 stimulates an appetite

79.
Orexi/mania means an abnormal desire (madness) for food or an uncontrollable appetite. What does orexi/genic mean? _____

_____.

orexigenic
ō rcks i gen´ ik

80.
Food that smells good and is appealing to the eye stimulates appetite. We may describe this food and its presentation as

_____.

anorexia
an o rek´ sē ə

81.
Along with malaise, loss of appetite is a very common symptom in many diseases. Write the term for loss of appetite. _____

82.
Complete each of the following definitions:

malaise

A vague sensation of not feeling well is _____.

nausea

Sickness of the stomach with a desire to vomit is _____.

emesis

Another word for vomitus is _____.

pyrexia

Elevated body temperature is _____.

anorexia

Loss of appetite is _____.

83.
A patient with an infection may experience a vague sensation of not feeling well. A patient with a fever may not have an appetite. When a fever and infection occur at the same time, the patient usually reports these two very subjective symptoms. What are they?

malaise
anorexia

_____ and _____.

84.
Anorexia and malaise are purely subjective symptoms. What does

the patient experiences
the sensation

that mean? _____

_____.

85.
Vertigo means a turning around. The patient experiences the sensation of turning around in space or having objects move about him.

86.
Vertigo is *not* dizziness, faintness, or lightheadedness. However, the patient may have difficulty maintaining equilibrium, and may

turning around

describe a sensation of spinning or _____ in space.

87.
An infection in the middle ear can cause a patient to experience the sensation of turning around in space or of objects moving about

symptom
vertigo
ver′ ti gō

her. This _____ is known as _____.
(sign/symptom)

88.
Tinnitus is a jingling, or tinkling, sound in the ear. It is often called ringing in the ear.

Toxicity or sensitivity to a drug like aspirin can cause ringing in

tinnitus
ti nī′ tus

the ear. Write the medical term for tinkling sound in the ear:

_____.

89.
Ménière's syndrome (pronounce ma nē ars′) is a recurrent and usually progressive group of symptoms including hearing loss, ringing in the ears, a sensation of fullness or pressure in the ears, and a turning around in space.

tinnitus

The term for ringing in the ears is _____.

vertigo

The sensation of turning about in space is _____.

90.

Try these and see how much you've learned. Select the best word from the suggested answers.

SUGGESTED ANSWERS:

erythroderma	leukocyte
melanoblast	cyanemia
chlorocyte	xanthemia

chlorocyte	green (plant) cell, _____.
xanthemia	yellowish blood, _____.
melanoblast	black (dark) immature cell, _____.
erythroderma	reddened skin, _____.
leukocyte	white blood cell, _____.
cyanemia	blue-bloodedness, _____.

91.

Now try these qualifiers.

hypertrophia	atrophy
general	systemic
local	

general or systemic	pertaining to the entire body _____.
hypertrophia	overdevelopment _____.
local	pertaining to a small area, or one part, _____.
systemic	pertaining to all body systems _____.
atrophy	a wasting away, underdevelopment, _____.

92.

Here are some objective symptoms.

tinnitus	malaise
emesis	nausea
vertigo	anorexia

vertigo	a sensation of turning around in space _____.
nausea	seasickness; inclined to vomit _____.
emesis	another word for vomitus _____.
tinnitus	ringing in the ears _____.
malaise	a vague sensation of not feeling well _____.
anorexia	loss of appetite _____.

Describing Illness

93.
A diagnosis is an identification of an illness. It requires scientific and skillful methods to establish the cause and nature of a sick person's disease. A diagnosis is arrived at by evaluating (a) the history of the person's disease, (b) the signs and symptoms present, (c) laboratory data, and (d) special tests such as X rays and electrocardiograms.

94.
In your English dictionary, you'll find words beginning with gnos. They come from the Greek word *gnosis,* meaning knowledge. *Dia* means through. Therefore, dia/gnosis literally means

knowing through _____.

95.
Diagnosing an illness means studying it through its signs and symptoms and other available information. When a patient reports chills, feels hot, and has a runny nose, the physician may identify the patient's illness as a head cold. This conclusion would be the

diagnosis
dī ag nō′ sis _____.

96.
A patient complains of pain in her arm after falling off her horse. An X ray shows a broken bone in her forearm. With this informa-
diagnosis tion from an X ray, the physician arrives at a _____.

identification of a
   patient's illness
   through blood
   (studies)

97.
What do you think hemodiagnosis means? _____
_____
_____.

98.
Many diseases are complex, so establishing the cause and nature of a sick person's disease requires skill and scientific methods. Which of the following might a physician use to help identify an illness? Check one or more.

all are relevant   _____ personal and family history
   _____ signs and symptoms
   _____ laboratory data
   _____ special tests, such as an X ray or ECG

one who is skilled in
making diagnoses

99.
If an obstetrician is one who is skilled in delivering babies, what is a
diagnostician? _____

_____.

(Here's our suggestion)
to predict the patient's
illness (its course and
outcome)

100.
The prefix pro- means before, or in front of. What do you think is
the meaning of prognosis? _____

_____

_____.

prognosis
prog nō′ sis

101.
Acute leukemia often may be fatal within three months. Prediction
of the course and outcome of this disease is called a _____.

to tell what the course
and likely outcome
of the disease will be

102.
What does prognosticate mean? _____

_____

_____.

103.
A prognosis predicts the course and outcome of a disease. Select a
term that best fits each outcome described.

favorable   unfavorable   guarded

unfavorable

Expect the patient to die in 3 to 6 months _____.

favorable

Recovery will be easy after surgery _____.

guarded

Recovery will be long and difficult _____.

unfavorable prognosis

104.
A patient who has little chance of recovering from his disease is said
to have an (two words) _____ _____.
                                unfavorable/favorable   predicted outcome

diagnosis

105.
When a physician has identified the patient's illness, the physician
has made a _____.

prognosis

106.
Prediction of the course and outcome of the disease is a

_____.

107.
A diagnosis may specify that the disease is acute, chronic, or paroxysmal.

Acute means sharp, severe, having a rapid onset and a short course,
not chronic.

paroxysm
par′ ok sizm
and
paroxysmal
par ok siz′ mal

Chronic means long, drawn out. A chronic disease is not acute.

Paroxysmal is from the Greek word *paroxysm*. It means a sudden
periodic attack or recurrence of symptoms of disease, a fit or convulsion of any kind.

chronic
kron′ ik

108.
Diabetes is a disease that has a long, drawn-out course. Therefore,
diabetes is a _____ disease.
                 (acute/chronic/paroxysmal)

paroxysmal
par ok sis′ mal

109.
Epilepsy is characterized by a sudden onset of symptoms that recur
periodically. Therefore, epilepsy is a _____ illness.
                                       (acute/chronic/paroxysmal)

suddenly recurring
    episode of difficult
    breathing

110.
Dys/pnea means difficult breathing. Paroxysmal dyspnea is another
way to describe asthma. Explain paroxysmal dyspnea. _____
_____
_____.

stomach
rapid

111.
Gastritis may be acute or chronic. Acute gastritis means inflammation of the _____. Its onset is _____,
                                                     (rapid/slow)

severe

the pain in the belly is _____, and the illness lasts a
                              (mild/severe)

short

_____ time.
        (short/long)

112.
A patient has a sudden onset of fast heart rate—in excess of 200
beats per minute—and then abruptly the heart rate returns to normal. This has occurred before. The diagnosis would be

paroxysmal tachy/cardia   _____ _____ / _____.
                          (acute/chronic/paroxysmal)   rapid   heart

113.
Arteriosclerotic heart disease (ASHD) has a very slow onset. Symptoms may be mild and last a lifetime. ASHD is a/an _____ condition.

chronic

114.
Inflammatory conditions may be either acute or chronic. Acute tendonitis means the tendon becomes red, hot, and very painful in a few hours. It returns to normal after a day or two of treatment.

inflammation that has a slow onset (may be mild) and lasts a long time

Describe chronic tendonitis: _____
_____
_____.

paroxysm
par′ ok sizm

115.
A fit or convulsion is a/an _____.

chronic

A long, drawn-out disease is described as _____.

acute

Sharp, severe symptoms, over a short course, describes a/an _____ disease.

116.
Poly- is a prefix meaning many or much; excessive. Explain each of the following:

an inflammation of many nerves, a rapid onset; very painful, short duration

Acute polyneuritis means _____
_____
_____.

an inflammation of many joints that starts slowly and lasts a long time

Chronic polyarthritis _____
_____
_____.

a condition of having supernumerary fingers (or toes)

Polydactylism _____
_____
_____.

117.
Syndrome is a group of symptoms that occur together and thus characterize a specific disease.

a group of symptoms running along together

Syn means together; *drome* means running along. Therefore, syndrome literally means _____
_____.

118.
For example, Korsakoff's syndrome is a psychosis, ordinarily due to chronic alcoholism. It is characterized by polyneuritis, disorientation, insomnia, muttering delirium, hallucinations, and a bilateral wrist or foot drop. Korsakoff's syndrome is characterized by this group of symptoms that occur _____.

together

119.
A syndrome is a variety of symptoms occurring together. When symptoms run along together, they present a complete picture of the disease. This is known as a _____.

syndrome
sin′ drōm

120.
Alcoholism produces a characteristic group of symptoms called Korsakoff's syndrome. From the name we know that a variety of _____ occur _____.

symptoms
together

121.
A group of symptoms occurring together characterize a specific disease. We call this group of symptoms a _____.

syndrome

122.
Recurrent (and usually progressive) hearing loss, tinnitus, vertigo, and a sensation of fullness in the ears is known as Ménière's _____.

syndrome

the symptoms run along together

Explain why: _____
_____.

123.
Pro/drome means running before (a disease). A symptom or group of symptoms may occur a few hours or a few days before the onset of the disease. These early signals are called its _____.

prodrome
prō′ drom

124.
The prodromal phase of a disease is the interval between the earliest symptoms and the appearance of a rash or fever. These symptoms occur _____ the onset of the disease.
(before/after)

before

125.
Sneezing that comes before the chills and fever of a common cold is the _____ of the cold.

prodrome

prodrom (al)
prō drō′ mal

126.
Malaise, anorexia, and sore throat occur one to four days before the fever and rash of measles appear. This early stage of the disease is called the _____al phase.

127.
It's time to review what you just covered. From the suggested answers, select the best term for each brief definition.

asymptomatic   acute
prognosis   prodromal
chronic   diagnose
syndrome   paroxysm

diagnose

to identify an illness, _____.

paroxysm

a sudden, recurrent attack, _____.

acute

pertaining to severe symptoms and rapid onset, _____.

prognosis

prediction of course and outcome of illness, _____.

syndrome

symptoms occurring together as a disease, _____.

asymptomatic

relating to symptom free, _____.

chronic

pertaining to a long, drawn-out illness, _____.

prodromal

earliest phase of signals and symptoms occurring before the onset of the fever or rash associated with a disease _____.

128.
Using scientific and skillful methods of investigation, a physician gathers information about a patient's illness in order to learn the cause and nature of a sick person's disease. Identification of the illness is called a _____.

diagnosis

Treatment

Treatment is the medical, surgical, or psychiatric management of a patient's illness. Although there are many different kinds of treatments, we're covering only a few of the most common.

129.
Active treatment aims for a cure. A patient suffering from appendicitis expects to be cured after an appendectomy. Since surgery removes the patient's appendix and usually cures the patient's disease, it is an _____ treatment.

active

active

130.
An antibiotic attacks the bacteria causing peritonitis. Therefore, antibiotic therapy is considered an _____ treatment.

systemic
sis tem′ ik

131.
Systemic treatment attacks constitutional signs and symptoms such as pyrexia, shock, and pain. Treatment directed toward control of these life-threatening signs is called _____ treatment.

life-threatening or
    constitutional

132.
Giving a patient morphine for pain is a systemic treatment that aims to relieve a _____ sign or symptom.

systemic

133.
Hyperpyrexia is a constitutional sign. Placing a hyperpyrexic child in a basin of ice water reduces the whole body temperature and is therefore a _____ treatment.

palliative
pal′ ē a tiv

134.
Palliative treatment relieves bothersome symptoms and makes a patient comfortable. Very little the physician can do alters the course of poison ivy dermatitis. The physician may suggest calamine lotion to reduce itching and burning, and therefore, calamine is called a _____ treatment.

prophylactic
prō fi lak′ tic

135.
Prophylaxis is a treatment modality that focuses on prevention of disease. Your dentist aims to prevent dental caries by applying flouride solution to your teeth. Flouride application is called a _____ treatment.

treatments

136.
Whether active, symptomatic, palliative, or prophylactic, things the physician does or prescribes to manage a patient's illness are called _____.

relieve symptoms

137.
Palliative treatment addresses a patient's comfort rather than attempting to cure the disease. The purpose of this kind of treatment is to _____.

cure
kyo͞or

138.
Active treatment squarely addresses the patient's pathological condition. The physician elects an active treatment modality when a remedy or therapy will _____ the disease.

139.
Shock, pyrexia, and pain are indications of disease, which if not treated could have very serious consequences. Systemic treatment is directed toward very serious constitutional signs of illness which may be _____.

life threatening

140.
From the terms listed, select one that best fits each description.

active   palliative
prophylactic   systemic

systemic

Treatment of constitutional symptoms, _____.

active

Treatment directed specifically toward a cure, _____.

palliative

Treatment to relieve discomfort, _____.

prophylactic

Treatment aimed at preventing disease, _____.

141.
There are many remedies and therapies a physician may use to treat a patient's illness. Here are a few of the major classes for you to investigate. Look up therapy in your medical dictionary.

pharmacotherapy   radiotherapy
physical therapy   electroshock therapy
chemotherapy   psychotherapy

Statistics

In medicine and health care, many people keep score. The Health and Human Services Agency (HHS) of the U.S. government and the World Health Organization (WHO) of the United Nations publish statistics showing how many people are affected by certain diseases and how many people die of their illnesses. In order to understand the statistics, there are two important terms to know: *morbidity* and *mortality*.

142.
Morbidity means a diseased state. A statistic that reports, "50 cases of measles per 10,000 people living in the United States last year" is called a _____ rate.

morbidity (or sickness)
mor bid′ i tē

143.
Mortality means the state of being mortal and, therefore, subject to death. In other words, mortality is a statistic that reports the _____ rate.

mortality (or death)
mor tal′ i tē

144.
Which of the following examples expresses a mortality rate? Check each correct example.

all three are mortality
statistics

a. _____ From 198X to 199X, 3 million people were killed in automobile accidents on U.S. highways.

b. _____ Hepatitis took the lives of 20 people of every 1,000 in Ethiopia in 198X.

c. _____ Thirty thousand children around the world died of leukemia in the last five years.

145.
The mortality rate is the same as saying the _____ rate.

death

146.
The morbidity rate is expressed as the number of cases of a specific disease found in a specific unit of population during a specific period of time. It shows the rate of _____.

sickness or disease

147.
Which of the following examples is a morbidity rate? Check each correct example.

a. reports rate of
sickness

a. _____ In 198X, there were 550 new cases of tuberculosis reported for every 100,000 people living in the United States.

b. _____ In 198X, there were 30 deaths from suicide for every 10,000 people between 35 and 55 years of age living in Colorado.

148.
A statistic that reports the number of cases of a disease in a specific population for a specific period of time is called _____ _____.

morbidity
rate

mortality
rate

149.
A statistic that reports the death rate is called _____
_____.

morbidity refers to the
rate of illness;
mortality refers to the
death rate

150.
What is the difference between a morbidity and a mortality statistic?
_____
_____
_____.

151.
In this unit you worked with many new terms and learned to use some familiar words in new ways. Fifty of these words are listed here for you to practice your pronunciation and to review their meanings. Pronounce each term, think about its meaning, and then take the Unit 7 Self-Test.

acute (a kūt′)
anorexia (an o rek′ sē ə)
antipyretic (an tē pī ret′ ik)
asymptomatic (ā simp tō mat′ ik)
atrophy (at′ rō fē)
bradypnea (brad′ ip nē ə)
central (sen′ trul)
Cheyne-Stokes respiration
  (chān-stōks)
chlorocyte (klor′ ō sīt)
chronic (kron′ ik)
cyanoderma (sī ə nō der′ mä)
diagnosis (dī ag nō′ sis)
dyspnea (disp′ nē ə)
edema (e dē′ mä)
emesis (em′ ə sis)
erythremia (er i thrē′ mē ə)
generalized
hematemesis (hē mä tem′ ə sis)
hyperpnea (h perp′ nē ə)
hyperpyrexia (hī per pī rek′ sē ə)
hypothermia (hī pō ther′ mē ə)
leukocyte (loo′ kō sīt)
localized
malaise (mä lāz′)
melanocarcinoma
  (mel′ ə no kar sin o′ ma)

morbidity (mor bid′ i tē)
mortality (mor tal′ i tē)
nausea (naw′ zē ə)
palliative (pal′ ē ə tiv)
paroxysmal (par ok sis′ mal)
peripheral (per i′ fer al)
pneometer (nē om′ ə ter)
polyarthritis (pol′ ē arth rī′ tis)
prodromal (prō drō′ mal)
prognosis (prog nō′ sis)
prophylactic (prō fi lak′ tic)
pulse (pultz′)
pyretolysis (pī ret ō lī′ sis)
pyrexia (pī rek′ sē ə)
respiration
symptom
symptomatic
syndrome (sin′ drōm)
systemic
tachypnea (tak ip nē′ ə)
temperature
tinnitus (ti nī′ tus)
vertigo (ver′ ti gō)
vital signs
xanthopsia (zan thop′ sē ə)

Unit 7: Self-Test

Part 1

From the list on the right, select the correct meaning for each of the following medical terms.

_____ 1. Diagnosis

_____ 2. Systemic

_____ 3. Morbidity

_____ 4. Pyretolysis

_____ 5. Edema

_____ 6. Generalized

_____ 7. Anorexia

_____ 8. Vertigo

_____ 9. Hyperpnea

_____ 10. Malaise

_____ 11. Paroxysm

_____ 12. Vital signs

_____ 13. Syndrome

_____ 14. Nausea

_____ 15. Atrophy

a. Pertaining to the whole body, all systems

b. Very fast breathing

c. Identification of an illness

d. Fluid in the tissues

e. Pertaining to disease rate statistic

f. Temperature, pulse, and respiration

g. Reduction of fever

h. A sickness of the stomach; desire to vomit

i. Pertaining to the whole body, many different parts at the same time

j. Wasting away, or underdevelopment

k. Loss of appetite

l. Sensation of turning around in space

m. Vague sensation of not feeling well

n. Pertaining to sudden periodic attack

o. Symptoms occurring together

Part 2

Complete each of the medical terms on the right with the appropriate missing part. Some terms are missing all parts!

1. Ringing in the ear   _____

2. Artery throbbing in time with the
   heartbeat   _____

3. Respiratory arrest, not breathing   _____

4. Outside surface of the body   _____

5. Pertaining to preventing disease   _____

6. Sudden recurring attack   _____

7. Symptom-free   _____

8. Breathing that reaches a climax, then
   ceases before beginning again   C_____-S_____
                                                                         respiration

9. Pertaining to relieving symptoms but
   not the disease   _____

10. Patient perceives change in body or
    functions   _____

11. Prediction of course and outcome of
    a disease   _____

12. Pertaining to severe symptoms, rapid
    onset, short course   _____

13. Reddened skin   _____

14. Subnormal body temperature
    under 90°F   _____

15. Feverishness   _____

ANSWERS

Part 1	Part 2
1. c	1. Tinnitus
2. a	2. Pulse
3. e	3. Apnea

4. g	4.	Peripheral
5. d	5.	Prophylactic
6. i	6.	Paroxysm
7. k	7.	Asymptomatic
8. l	8.	Cheyne-Stokes respiration
9. b	9.	Palliative
10. m	10.	Symptom
11. n	11.	Prognosis
12. f	12.	Acute
13. o	13.	Erythroderma
14. h	14.	Hypothermia
15. j	15.	Pyrexia

8 Growth and Development, and Body Orientation

In this unit you will work with terms relating to growth and development of an embryo and other kinds of growing things. You'll cover terms that provide an orientation to the body, something like a road map, to make anatomical descriptions meaningful.

Mini-Glossary

cyst	benign	distal
lesion	infiltration	dorsal
polyp	malignant	lateral
papilla	metastasis	medial
papilloma	neoplasm	proximal
papule		ventral

ecto-, exo- (outer side)

end-, endo- (inner, within)

meso- (middle)

circum- (around)

peri- (around about)

epi- (over, surrounding)

sub-, hypo- (below, under)

supra-, super- (above, over)

infra- (below, beneath)

Have you completed the Section 7 Review Sheet? We suggest you do it before you begin. It will really help you learn.

Growth and Development

1.

Blastos refers to a germ, seed, sprout, or bud. A *blastoderm* is an aggregation of cells showing the first trace of structure in a microscopic organism. It is the most rudimentary form of a developing embryo and is made up of three primary germ cell layers: the *ectoderm, endoderm,* and *mesoderm.* From these primordial germ layers the embryo develops and becomes a fetus.

2.

Review these definitions and return to them as you need help with the frames that follow.

Ectoderm is the outer layer of cells in the primary germ layers of the developing embryo. It is the origin of:

- the skin (epidermis)

- the mucous membranes of nose, mouth, and anus (epithelium)

- nervous tissue and sensory organs

Mesoderm is the middle of the three primary germ layers of the embryo. It is the origin of:

- all connective tissues

- all body musculature

- blood, cardiovascular and lymphatic systems

- most of the urogenital system

- the lining of the pericardial, pleural, and peritoneal cavities

Endoderm is the innermost of the three primary germ layers of the embryo, from which are derived:

- the lining of the gut

- its glands (spleen, pancreas, liver)

- component structures of the gut (esophagus, stomach, intestine, colon)

- the respiratory tract

3.

Ectoderm is the outer layer of cells. Endoderm is the innermost of the three germ layers. Mesoderm is the middle layer of three primary germ layers in the developing embryo. Write a meaning for each of the prefixes:

inner, inside   endo- means _____.

middle   meso- means _____.

outer, outside   ecto- means _____.

4.

mesoderm   Which primary germ layer originates all connective tissues and all
mēz′ ō derm   body musculature? _____.

5.

                  The pleura is a watery, mucoid-surfaced membrane enveloping the
                  lungs and lining the walls of the thoracic cavity. From which germ
mesoderm   layer does it arise? _____.

6.

ectoderm   Which of the three embryonic germ layers gives rise to the nervous
ek′ tō derm   system and the organs of special sense? _____.

7.

endoderm   The primative gut tract and its associated glands (organs) develop
en′ dō derm   from which germ layer of the embryo? _____.

8.

                  The skin, including mucous membranes exposed to the environ-
                  ment, is derived from the primary germ layer called the

ectoderm   _____.

9.

endoderm   The innermost of the three primary germ layers of the embryo is
ectoderm   the _____. The outside layer of cells in the embryo
mesoderm   is the _____. The middle of the three primary
mēz′ ō derm   germ layers is the _____.

10.

                  Now let's try out those new prefixes. Write a meaning for each of
                  the following:

of, or pertaining to   ectocytic _____
   outside the cell
                         _____.

inflammation of inside of the heart	endocarditis _____ _____.
examination by looking inside of (a body cavity)	endoscopy _____ _____.
examination of inside the bladder	endocystoscopy _____ _____.

11.

Gen/o is the combining form to denote originating or production.

Ectogenous means originating outside of a cell or an organism. Underline the part of the term meaning originating or produced.

ecto<u>genous</u> ek toj' en us	Ectogenous
originating or produced inside of (a cell) en doj' en us	What does endogenous mean? _____ _____

12.

Topos, top/o means place or location. Sometimes a pregnancy begins in the fallopian tube instead of within the uterus. It is called an ectopic pregnancy.

pregnancy outside of its normal location	What is an ectopic pregnancy? _____ _____.

13.

ectopic ek top' ik	A pregnancy beginning in the abdominal cavity instead of the womb is called an _____ pregnancy.

14.

Let's review before going on. From the suggested answers, select the best term for each brief definition.

SUGGESTED ANSWERS:

ecto-, exo-	endo-, en-, end-
ectopic	endocranial
ectocytic	endogenous
meso-	mesoderm

ecto- (exo-)	outside (prefix), _____.
meso-	middle (prefix), _____.
endo- (en- or end-)	inside (prefix), _____.

mesoderm	middle germ cell layer, _____.
endogenous	originating inside, _____.
ectocytic	pertaining to outside the cell, _____.
ectopic	out of its normal place, _____.
endocranial	pertaining to inside the head, _____.

Growths and Other Abnormal Tissues

15.

In this section you'll work with more terms relating to growth. Growing means to increase progressively in size. However, growth may be normal and purposeful, or abnormal and useless. Here are some terms used to describe abnormal growth.

16.

Neo- means new; *-plasm* means thing formed. Neoplasm is a new formation of tissue. It is abnormal because it serves no useful function and grows at the expense of a healthy body. Any tissue growing autonomously and that has no useful function is a _____.

neoplasm
nē′ ō plazm

17.

A tumor is a swelling or enlargement. It is an autonomous new growth of tissue. It is a mass of tissue without a function. Another word for tumor is _____.

neoplasm

18.

Neoplasm and tumor are interchangeable terms. They both mean an autonomous new _____ _____.

growth of tissue that
serves no useful
purpose

19.

Bio- means life; *-opsy* means appearance, sight. A biopsy is removing tissue from a living body and examining it under a microscope.

To make a diagnosis, a physician usually biopsies a tumor or neoplasm. This means the physician removes a piece of living _____ and _____ it under a microscope.

tissue
examines

20.

A neoplasm (tumor) growing in or on the human body can be classified as either malignant or benign.

Malignant means it's of a bad kind, growing worse, resisting treatment, and tending or threatening to produce death.

benign
bē nīn′
malignant
ma lig′ nant

Benign means it's mild (grows slowly), not spreading, not recurrent, and not malignant. Tumors may be of uncertain behavior, but usually are classified either as _____ or _____.

21.
To determine what kind of neoplasm a patient has, the physician removes a piece of the living tumor tissue and examines it under a microscope. What is this procedure called? _____.

biopsy

22.
A biopsy report indicates a patient's abnormal growth is of a bad kind. It will grow worse (rapidly), resist treatment, and tend to be life-threatening. The diagnosis is _____ neoplasm.
                                                    (malignant/benign)

malignant

23.
A nonmalignant neoplasm is an abnormal tissue mass growing slowly, not spreading, and not likely to recur. The growth is

benign

_____.
(malignant/benign)

24.
A procedure that determines whether a neoplasm is benign or malignant is a _____.

biopsy

25.
A malignant neoplasm is a bad kind that grows _____,
                                                    (fast/slowly)

fast

death

resists treatment, and threatens to cause _____.

26.
A benign neoplasm is mild (grows slowly), does not spread or recur, and is not _____.
                              (the other kind)

malignant

27.
Infiltration means slipping into and between normal cells of the body.

Malignant tumor cells may spread by slipping into and between normal body cells. Malignant cells multiply rapidly and take up nourishment and space, crowding out the normal cells. This method of spreading is called direct extension or _____.

infiltration

28.
Metastasis means movement of cells (especially cancer cells) from one part of the body to another.

Meta- means after, beyond, among, over; *-stasis* means a standing, a location, or place.

metastasis
me tas′ tə sis

Malignant tumor cells migrate to another location and take up a standing in another organ or part of the body. This method of spreading the disease is called invasion by _____.

29.

location

Metastasis is the movement of malignant tumor cells from the primary location over to another _____.

30.

infiltration or direct extension

metastasis

There are two methods by which a malignant neoplasm spreads, grows larger, and becomes more threatening. Malignant cells may slip into and between normal cells. This is called _____ _____. Or tumor cells may move beyond the primary site and take up a standing in another location of the body. This spreading method is called _____.

31.

infiltration
metastasis

Unlike malignant neoplasms, benign growths do not spread by _____ or _____.

32.
Here's a quick review. Select a term from the suggested answers that best fits each brief definition. Write your selection in the space provided.

malignant neoplasm/tumor
tumor/neoplasm biopsy
benign infiltration
metastasize

biopsy

remove tissue for examination, _____.

benign

slow growth, not malignant, _____.

neoplasm/tumor

new, abnormal tissue mass, _____.

tumor/neoplasm

tissue mass, no useful purpose, _____.

malignant

fast-growing, threatening death, _____.

infiltration

slipping into and between normal cells, _____.

metastasize
(me tās′ tə sīz)

cells relocate to new location, organ, _____.

33.
There are many other terms that mean abnormal conditions, changes, or growths. Here are a few of the more common ones.

34.
Lesion is an area of unhealthy (morbid) tissue, such as an injury, wound, burn, or infected patch of skin.

lesion
lē′ zhun

Any morbid change in the structure of an organ or a body part due to injury or disease is called a _____.

35.
An infected finger is a lesion because there has been a morbid change in the finger tissues. What does morbid mean?

diseased, unhealthy

_____.

36.
In Alzheimer's disease there are morbid changes in brain tissue. These unhealthy changes in brain structure are also called _____.

lesions

37.
An injury, a burn, and an infected finger are examples of lesions because the part of the body involved has undergone a _____ change.

morbid

(unhealthy)

38.
A lesion is any morbid change in the structure of an organ or part due to injury or disease. Check each item that is *not* a lesion.

☒ chicken pox is a
disease; the pox are
lesions

☐ duodenal ulcer
☐ skinned knees
☐ scalding burn of the hand
☐ abrasion of the elbow
☐ chicken pox
☐ infected toenail

39.
Poison ivy leaves may irritate the skin and cause blisters. These unhealthy changes in the structure of the skin are called _____.

lesions

40.
Build a word meaning a hurt, an injury, or any unhealthy area of
any organ or part: _____.

lesion

41.
What does morbid mean? _____.

unhealthy, diseased

42.
In earlier units you learned that cyst means bladder.

inflammation of the
    bladder

Cystitis means _____
_____.

examination of the
    inside of the bladder

Endocystoscopy means _____
_____
_____.

excision (or removal) of
    the gallbladder

Cholecystectomy means _____
_____
_____.

43.
Cyst also means a closed sac or pouch that contains fluid, semifluid,
or solid material.

sac

A cyst is a closed _____.

fluid, semifluid, or solid
    material

It contains _____
_____.

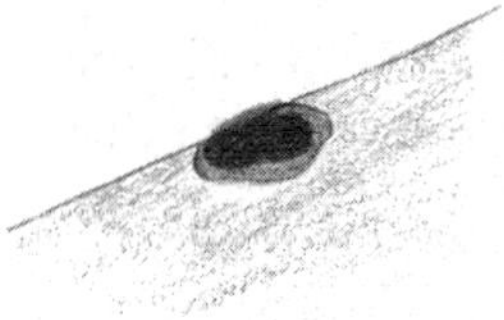

Figure 8.1   Cyst

44.
A malfunctioning ovary may develop a closed sac or pouch containing fluid. This is called an ovarian _____.

cyst

45.
What is a hydrocyst? _____
_____.

a cyst containing fluid
    (water)

a sac that contains fluid
    or even solid material

Cyst means _____
_____.

46.
A physician doesn't usually drain a cyst of its contents because it only would fill again. Instead, a surgeon completely excises the cyst. Write

cystectomy
a term meaning surgical removal of a cyst: _____.

47.

pol′ ip
Polyp is a tumor with a little foot, or stem. A polyp is usually a

malignant
benign tumor. That means it is not _____,
(the other kind)

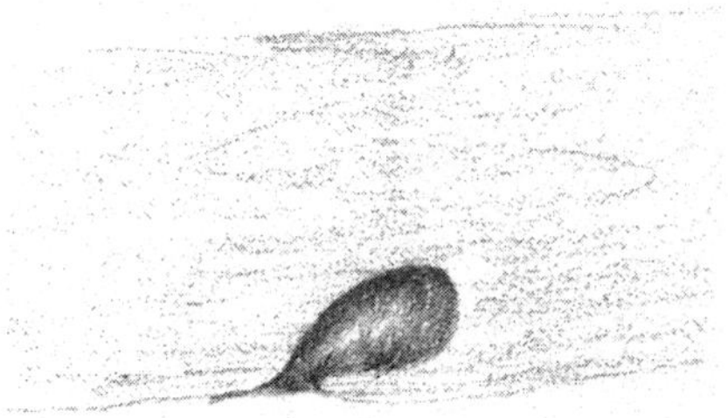

Figure 8.2   Polyp.

slowly
it grows _____, and it does *not* spread by
(fast/slowly)

infiltration

metastasis
_____ or _____.

48.
A polyp is a specific type of tumor or neoplasm. It's an abnormal,

foot
useless new growth that stands on a stem or a little _____.

49.
Vascular organs such as the nose, uterus, and rectum commonly develop polyps. Polyps bleed easily and usually are removed surgi-

polypectomy
cally. Build a word for excision of polyps: _____.

What does vascular mean? This is a good time to use your dictionary.

_____

50.

unhealthy
A lesion is an area of _____ tissue.

Give some examples of lesions: _____

burn, injury, infection
_____.

51.
Cyst has two different meanings.

bladder

Cyst means _____.
a part of the body

a sac containing fluid or
  semifluid

Cyst also means _____.
an abnormality

52.

tumor/neoplasm
little foot, or stem

A polyp is a specific kind of _____.
A polyp has a _____.

53.
Papilla is a small nipplelike protuberance or elevation. It may be
located anywhere on the body, and may be normal or abnormal.

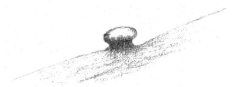

Figure 8.3   Papilla.

Taste buds are small nipplelike structures on the surface of the
tongue. They account for the four fundamental taste sensations:
sweet, bitter, sour, and salt. Stand in front of a mirror; stick your
tongue way out. You will see papillae (plural) on the back of your
tongue. Describe them: _____.

small, nipplelike
  structures

54.

papilla
pa pil′ ə

The nipple of the mammary gland (breast) is called a mammary
_____.

55.

pap i lō′ mä

Papilloma is a hypertrophied papilla covered by a layer of skin. What
is the shape of a papilloma?

nipplelike

_____.

56.

pap′ yōol

Papule is a pimple. It's a red elevated spot on the skin. It's solid and
circumscribed. Papular lesions appear on the skin in smallpox,
measles, and chicken pox.

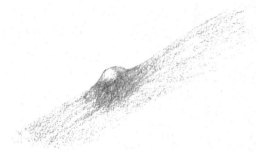

Figure 8.4   Papule.

spots

circumscribed

They are elevated red _____ on the skin.

They are solid and _____.

57.
Excrescence: ex means out; *crescence* means to grow. Excrescence is a useless structure growing out of the surface of a part such as a wart or mole.

The Wicked Witch of the West had a big wart growing on the tip of her nose. A medical term for this disfiguring outgrowth is

excrescence
eks kres′ ens

_____.

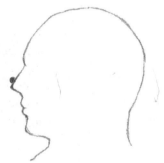

Figure 8.5   Excrescence.

58.
Condyloma is a wartlike growth of the skin, usually occurring near the anus. The main difference between an excrescence and a condyloma is where the lesion is located. An excrescence may appear anywhere on the surface of the body (even on the end of your nose). But a wartlike skin growth near the anus is called a _____.

kon di lō′ mä
condyloma

59.
An excrescence, a papilloma, a condyloma, and a papule are all lesions of the skin. That means the area of the skin involved is considered _____.

morbid, unhealthy

pa pil′ ē (pl.)
small, nipplelike
    protuberance

60.
Papillae (plural) may be normal structures on the body that have important functions. A taste bud is a papilla. Describe what it looks like: _____.

(For help in learning the plural forms, see Appendix B: *Forming Plurals.*)

61.
Label each of the following illustrations.

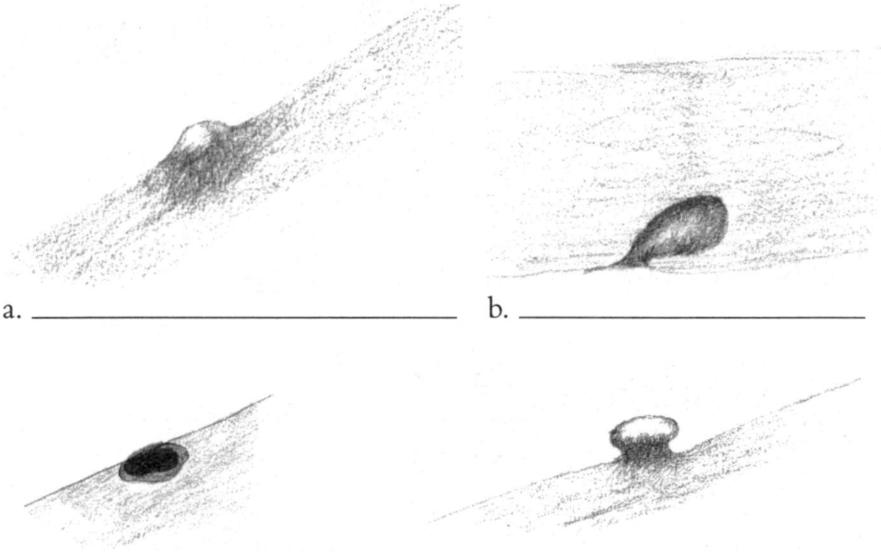

a. papule
b. polyp

a. _____   b. _____

c. cyst
d. papilloma

c. _____   d. _____

Figure 8.6

62.
Complete each definition.

SUGGESTED ANSWERS
papillae   condyloma
excrescence   lesion
polyp   papule
cyst

lesion (lē′ zhun)   area of unhealthy (morbid) tissue, _____.
polyp (pol′ ip)   tumor on a stem or little foot, _____.
condyloma   wartlike growth around the anus, _____.
    (kon di lō′ mä)

cyst (sist) | bladder, or a closed sac with fluid, _____.
excrescence (eks kres′ ens) | useless outgrowth, like a wart, _____.
papillae (pa pil′ ē) | nipplelike protuberances, _____.
papule (pap′ yōol) | small, elevated red lesion on the skin, _____.

63.
Here's an independent learning exercise for you. These are words related to treatments and consequences of malignant neoplasms. Look up each one in your medical dictionary. Explore it thoroughly; pronounce it several times. Then write a brief definition for each. Do this exercise even if you think you know what the terms mean. Sometimes you'll be surprised!

abdominal paracentesis

_____

_____

alopecia

_____

_____

anastomosis

_____

_____

cauterization

_____

_____

chemotherapy

_____

_____

dehiscence

_____

_____

necrobiosis

_____

_____

radiation

_____

_____

radical resection

_____

_____

Orientation

64.

Neoplasms, cysts, and lesions occur anywhere on the surface of the body and inside, under, and around organs and structures. Physicians use specific terms to describe where lesions and other morbid conditions are located relative to parts of the body.

65.

Ventral means on or near the belly, or the side of the body where the belly is located.

back

Dorsal is the opposite of ventral; it means on or near the _____.

Label the illustrations.

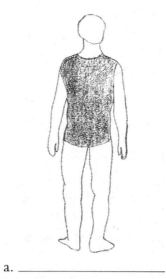
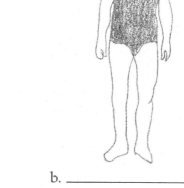

a. dorsal
b. ven′ tral
   ven′ tral

a. _____   b. _____

Figure 8.7

66.

belly
back

Ventral, ventr/o means on or near the _____. Dorsal, dors/o means on or near the _____.

67.
Try these.

backache   Dorsalgia means _____.

incision into the belly   Ventrotomy means _____.

68.
of or pertaining to belly   What do you think ventrodorsad means? _____
to back   _____.

                              A bullet penetrated the abdominal wall, traveled through the belly,
ventrodorsad   and exited through the back. The bullet's path may be described as
ven trō dor′ säd   _____.

69.
The *midline,* or median, is an imaginary line dividing the body into
right and left halves.

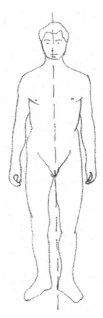

Figure 8.8   Midline of the Body.

Lateral means farther from the midline.

Medial means the opposite.

nearer   Medial means _____ to the midline.

                              Which is nearer the midline, your shoulder or your nipple?
nipple   _____.

70.

lateral

Which corner of your eye is nearest your ear? _____.
(medial/lateral)

medial

Which side of your knee knocks the other knee? _____.
(medial/lateral)

71.

farther

Lateral means _____ from the midline.

nearer

Medial means _____ to the midline.

on the midline

Where is your umbilicus located? _____.

72.

Let's describe a relative position in another way. *Distal* means remote, or farthest, from the point of attachment to the trunk.

nearest

Proximal means the opposite. Proximal means _____ to
(farthest/nearest)

the point of attachment to the trunk.

73.

hand

Which is distal, your elbow or your hand? _____.

proximal

On which end of your finger do you wear a ring? _____.
(distal/proximal)

74.

Your forearm bone has two ends. Your hand is attached to the

distal

_____ end.
(distal/proximal)

proximal

Your upper arm is located on the _____ end.
(distal/proximal)

75.

A part of the body located nearest its attachment to the trunk is

proximal

described as _____.

A part located farthest from its attachment to the trunk is described

distal

as _____.

76.

farthest from the
attachment to the
trunk

The fingers are distal to all other parts of the arm. What does distal mean? _____
_____.

nearest to the
attachment to the
trunk

77.
Describe the location of a part that is proximal:

_____

_____.

78.
Here's a review of what you just covered. Select the best term from the suggested answers to complete each definition.

SUGGESTED ANSWERS:
distal   proximal
medial   lateral
ventral   midline
dorsal

dorsal   near, or on the back, _____.

ventral   near, or on the belly, _____.

midline   divides body into right and left halves, _____.

lateral   farther from the midline, _____.

medial   nearer to the midline, _____.

distal   farthest from the attachment to the trunk, _____.

proximal   nearest to the attachment to the trunk, _____.

79.
Here are some prefixes indicating place or relative position:

Peri-, circum- means around, about, surrounding,

Write a meaning for each of the following:

pertaining to around
the tonsil

Peri/tonsillar _____

_____.

relating to around the
belly button

Peri/umbilical _____

_____.

80.
diseased (unhealthy)
tissue around the
teeth

What is peri/dent/al (peri/dont/al) gum disease? _____

_____

_____.

around   Peri– means _____.

81.

around

Circum- is another prefix meaning _____. *Duct/ion* means moving.

moving around

Ab/duct/ion is moving away. Circum/duction means _____ _____.

82.

circum(-scribed)

A wheal (hives) is a round patch of unhealthy skin with a ring of normal tissue at its circumference. A wheal appears as a round red spot. We usually say a wheal is _____-scribed.

83.

circumscribed

A boil also has an outer limit where the circumference of the lesion becomes normal. Because it appears to have a border around its circumference, you may also describe a boil as a _____ lesion.

84.

relating to around the mouth

Perioral and circumoral have the same meaning. Write the meaning: _____.

pertaining to around or surrounding the kidney

Write a meaning for circumrenal, perirenal:

_____

_____.

85.

Look over the following terms and their meanings and then complete the frames that follow. Come back to this frame whenever you need help.

Epi-	upon, over (surrounding or covering)
Extra-	without, outside of
Infra-	below, beneath, under
Sub-, hypo-	below, beneath, less than normal
Supra-, super-	above, superior, in the upper part of

86.

The epi/gastric region is the region of the belly over or upon the stomach. Refer to Illustration 8.9.

pain in the area of the belly over the stomach

Epi/gastralgia means _____

_____

_____.

hernia in the area of the belly over the stomach	Epi/gastrocele means _____ _____ _____.
	87. Epi/cranium refers to the tissues (muscle and skin) that cover and surround the cranium. What do you think epi/dermis means? _____
the skin (that covers the entire body)	_____.
	88. Again refer to the definitions in Frame 85. The prefix extra- means
without, outside of	_____.
outside the uterus	Extra/uterine means _____
outside the edges or outer limits of a structure or organ	Extra/marginal means _____ _____ _____.
	89. Again use the definitions to help you. The prefix *infra-* means
below, beneath, under	_____.
pertaining to an area under, below the kneecap	*Patella* means kneecap. What does infra/patellar mean? _____ _____.
beneath, under the kneecap	Sub/patellar means _____ _____.
	90. Infra- and sub- usually are interchangeable terms. Complete the alternate terms and write a meaning:
infra (–mammary)	_____–mammary
sub (–mammary)	_____–mammary
below the breast	meaning _____.
	91. Sub- and hypo- are often interchangeable also. Sub/lingual means
under the tongue	_____.
	Hypo/glossal means
under the tongue	_____.

92.

below, beneath, less than normal

The prefix sub- means _____ _____. What other two prefixes often are interchangeable and mean the same thing as sub- ? _____ and

infra-,
hypo-

_____.

93.

Sternum is the breastbone. Write a meaning for sub/sternal:

pertaining to below the breastbone

_____

_____.

Use another prefix and build another term that means the same

infrasternal

thing: _____.

94.

Build a term that means pertaining to above the sternum:

suprasternal

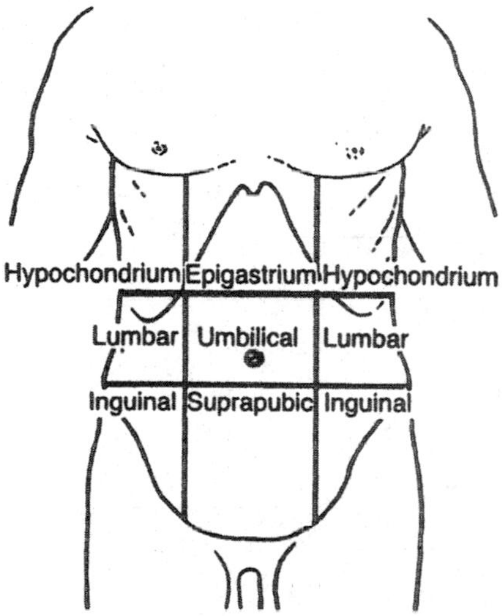

_____.

Figure 8.9   Regions of the Abdomen

95.

Refer to Illustration 8.9 to help you complete the next few frames.

96.

Sub/pubic refers to an area beneath the pubic arch (bone). Build a term meaning relating to the area above the pubic arch:

suprapubic

_____.

umbilicus or belly button

Umbilical is the term meaning relating to the area that is near/ around the _____.

beneath the ribs (These floating ribs are composed mostly of cartilage)	97. Chondros means cartilage (of ribs). Literally, hypochondrium means the area _____.
inguinal ing' gwi nal	98. Look at Illustration 8.9, Regions of the Abdomen. Lumbar relates to the loin. It is the part of the back and sides between the ribs and the pelvis. What area is below the lumbar region? _____.
	99. Write a meaning for each of the following terms.
pertaining to around the umbilicus	Peri/umbilical, _____ _____.
relating to below the abdomen	Sub/abdominal, _____ _____.
relating to above the loin	Supra/lumbar, _____ _____.
pertaining to below the pubic arch	Infra/pubic, _____ _____.
pertaining to around the intestine	Circum/intestinal, _____ _____.
pertaining to under the skin	Hypo/dermic, _____ _____.
relating to outside the field of vision	Extra/visual, _____ _____.
pertaining to over the stomach	Epigastric _____ _____

100.
In this unit you worked with 36 new medical terms. Practice pronouncing them. Then take the Unit 8 Self-Test.

benign (bē nīn')	dorsal
biopsy	ectoderm (ek tō derm)
circumocular	ectopic (ek top' ik)
circumscribed	endocystoscopy
condyloma (kon di lō' mä)	(en dō sis tos' ko pē)
cyst (sist)	endogenous (en doj' ə nus)
distal	epigastric (ep ē gas' trik)

excrescence (eks kres′ ens)

extrasensory (eks tra sen′ sō rē)

hypodermic (hī pō derm′ ik)

infiltration

inframammary (in fra mam′ ə rē)

lateral

lesion

lumbar

malignant (ma lig′ nant)

medial

mesoderm (mēz′ ō derm)

metastasis (me tas′ ta sis)

neoplasm (nē ō plazm)

papilla (pa pil′ ə)

papilloma (pap i lō′ mä)

papules (pap′ yōols)

periumbilical
    (per′ ē um bil′ i k'l)

polyp (pol′ ip)

proximal (prox′ si mal)

subpatellar (sub pa tel′ ar)

suprapubic (su pra pyōo′ bik)

tumor

ventral

Unit 8 Self-Test

Part 1

From the right, select the correct meaning for each of the following often used medical terms.

_____ 1. Endocystoscopy	a. Farthest point from trunk attachment
_____ 2. Lesion	
_____ 3. Circumocular	b. Outside layer of germ cells
_____ 4. Distal	c. Not spreading, not malignant
_____ 5. Endocranial	d. Pertaining to inside the head vault
_____ 6. Epigastric	e. Pertaining to around the eye
_____ 7. Biopsy	f. Slipping into and between normal cells
_____ 8. Neoplasm	
_____ 9. Ectoderm	g. Pertaining to the area over the stomach
_____ 10. Metastasis	h. Cells spread to new location, organ
_____ 11. Malignant	i. Removal of tissue for examination
_____ 12. Benign	j. New, abnormal tissue formation
_____ 13. Infiltration	k. Morbid tissue
_____ 14. Proximal	l. Nearest the attachment to the trunk
_____ 15. Ectopic	m. A bad kind, tending to threaten death
	n. Occurring outside the normal place
	o. Examination inside the bladder

Part 2

Write the medical term for each of the following brief definitions.

1. Nipplelike protuberance _____

2. New, abnormal tissue without a purpose _____

3. Useless structure growing out of the skin (wart) _____

4. Spread of cells to new location, organ _____

5. Pertaining to on or near the back _____

6. Farthest point from trunk attachment _____

7. Closed sac or pouch containing fluid _____

8. Removal of tissue for examination _____

9. Wartlike growth around the anus Con_____

10. Slipping into and between normal cells _____

11. Not spreading, not malignant _____

12. Below the mammary gland _____

13. Tumor with a little foot _____

14. Nearest point of trunk attachment _____

15. Unhealthy, diseased area of tissue _____

ANSWERS

Part 1	*Part 2*
1. o	1. Papilla
2. k	2. Neoplasm/tumor
3. e	3. Excrescence
4. a	4. Metastasis
5. d	5. Dorsal
6. g	6. Distal
7. i	7. Cyst
8. j	8. Biopsy
9. b	9. Condyloma

10. h	10. Infiltration
11. m	11. Benign
12. c	12. Inframammary
13. f	13. Polyp
14. l	14. Proximal
15. n	15. Lesion

9 Gynecology, Pregnancy, and Childbirth

This unit covers medical terms used in gynecology, pregnancy, and childbirth. This lesson may be difficult at times, so be kind to yourself and go slowly. If you don't get the right answers the first time you work through a sequence, try again before moving on. Here are the whole terms, word roots, prefixes, and suffixes you'll work with.

Mini-Glossary

-ary (*of or pertaining to*)

-atrophy (*undernourished, wasting*)

-dynia (*pain, painful*)

-mania (*madness*)

-pathy (*disease*)

-phobia (*excessive fear*)

primi- (*first*)
secundi- (*second*)
nulli- (*none*)
multi- (*many*)

climacteric
conception
embryo

amni/o, amniot/o (*fetal sac*)

gravid/a (*with child*)

gyn/o, gynec/o (*woman*)

hyster/o (*uterus*)

mamm/o (*breast*)

mast/o (*breast*)

men/o (*menses, menstruation*)

metr/o (*uterus*)

para (*bear, bring forth*)

pre- (*before*)
post- (*after*)
oligo- (*little, small, scanty*)

episiotomy
fetus
gestation

involution	perineum
labor	peritoneum
menopause	placenta
ovum	pudenda
parturition	puerperium

Do yourself a big favor. Complete the Review Sheet for Unit 8 before you tackle this unit.

Terms of Gynecology

1.

women

Gyn, gynec/o means woman. Gynecology is the study of the female reproductive organs and breasts. Simply put, it is the field of medicine dealing with diseases of whom? _____.

Before continuing, go to Illustration 4.2, The Female Reproductive Organs. Review the illustration and read again the description that follows.

2.

gī′ nō plas tē or jin′ ō plas tē
plastic surgery of female reproductive organs

Gyn/o/pathic means pertaining to diseases of female reproductive organs. What do you think gyn/o/plasty means? _____

_____

_____ .

3.

gī ne fo′ bē a
fear of women

Mania means madness. *Phobia* means excessive fear. Gynecomania is an abnormal sex drive and desire in the male of the species. What do you think gyne/phobia means? _____ .

4.

gynecologist
gī ne kol′ ō jist

The physician who specializes in female disorders is called a

_____ .

5.

breast

Human beings are mammals. Mammals have glands that secrete milk for nourishing their offspring. In plain English, mammary gland refers to _____ .

6.

These next two terms often are interchangeable. However, we use one term more often than the other. In this lesson you'll be using the *preferred terms.* Let's see what this means:

breast

Mamm, mamm/o refers to mammary gland, or breast; mast, mast/o also refers to _____.

mam ī′ tis,
mast ī′ tis
inflammation of the
    mammary gland
    (breast)
preferred

7.
Mamm/itis and mast/itis both mean

_____

_____.

Mastitis is the term used most often, so we say it is the
_____ term.

ma mog′ ra fē
mamm/o/graphy
X ray exam of the
    breast

8.
Break down each of the following preferred terms and write its meaning.

Mammography, _____ / ____ / _____
means _____

_____

mas tek′ tō mē
mast/ectomy
surgical removal of a
    breast

Mastectomy, _____ / _____
means _____

_____.

9.
Using the word root or combining form, mast, mast/o, add a suffix from the list and build a preferred term. Write its meaning in the space provided.

-otomy   -itis   -pathy

mastotomy
mas tot′ ō mē
incision into the breast

M _____
means _____

_____;

mastitis
inflammation of the
    breast

m _____
means _____

_____;

mastopathy
mas top′ a thē
disease of the
    mammary gland

m _____
means _____

_____.

10.
Very large breasts that hang down, or droop, are described as pendulous. The suffix for hanging or drooping is -ptosis. Construct a word meaning pendulous breast: _____.

mastoptosis
mas top tō′ sis

gī ne kō mas′ tē a
woman's breast

11.

Here's an interesting term that doesn't follow the rules. Let's look at the parts. Gynec/o means woman; mastia means breast.

Gynecomastia literally means _____.

In actual use it means abnormally large mammary glands in the male; sometimes they secrete milk.

12.

This time use mamm, mamm/o. Build a term with each of the following suffixes and write its meaning:

mam′ ō gram
mammogram
X ray picture of the
  breast

–gram   –ary

M _____

means _____

_____;

mam′ a rē
mammary
pertaining to the
  mammary gland

m _____

means _____

_____.

mam′ ō plas tē
plastic surgery of the
  mammary gland

13.

Mamm/o/pexy means surgical correction (fixation) of large hanging breasts. What does mamm/o/plasty mean? _____

_____

mast′ ad nī tis
mast′ ad nō′ ma
tumor of the mammary
  gland

14.

Mast/aden/itis means inflammation of the mammary gland. Write a meaning for each of the following:

mastadenoma _____

_____;

mas tō kar cin ō′ ma
cancerous tumor of the
  mammary gland

mastocarcinoma _____

_____.

mas tong′ kus
(any) tumor of the
  breast

15.

The study or science dealing with the physical, chemical, and biologic properties of neoplasms including causation, pathogenesis, and treatment is oncology. What does mastoncus mean? _____

_____.

mast/algia
mast al′ jē ə

16.
Mast/o/dynia means painful breast. Using another suffix you know, build another word that also means pain in the breast: mast/_____.

17.
Here's a quick review. Select a term from the suggested answers that best fits each brief definition. Write your selection in the space provided.

mastectomy	mastopathy
mastoptosis	gynecomastia
mastoncus	mastopexy

mastopathy
mas top′ a thē

disease of the mammary glands, _____.

gynecomastia

women's breasts (on a man), _____.

mastectomy

surgical removal of the breast, _____.

mastoptosis

pendulous breasts, _____.

mastoncus

any tumor of the breast, _____.

mastopexy
mas′ tō pex′ sē

surgical fixation of pendulous breasts, _____.

18.
Now try these.

mammoplasty	mammary
mammology	mammalgia (mastodynia)
mammography	gynecophobia

mammography

X ray study of the breast, _____.

mammalgia
(mastodynia)

painful breast, _____.

mammology

science and study of the breast, _____.

gynecophobia

fear of women, _____.

mammary

pertaining to the breast, _____.

mammoplasty

surgical reconstruction of the breast, _____.

19.
Mamma mē′ a, you're doing very well!

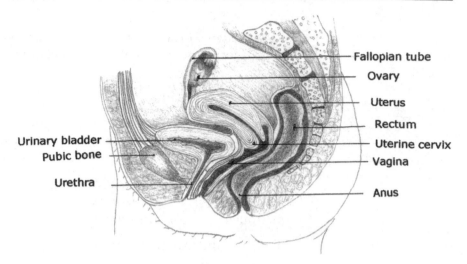

Figure 9.1   The Female Reproductive Organs (Midline Section).

See Illustration 4.2 for a description of The Female Reproductive System.

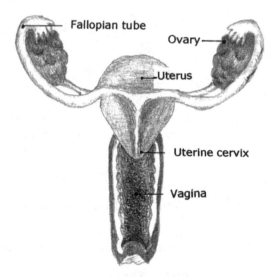

Figure 9.2   The Female Reproductive Organs (Anterior View).

ovary (oophor/o)   breast (mamm/o, mast/o)
fallopian tube (salping/o)   menses (men/o)
uterus (hyster/o, metr/o)   muscle (my/o)
uterine cervix (cerv/i)   bladder (cyst/o)
vagina (vagin/o)   urethra (urethr/o)

20.
Here are two more terms with nearly identical meanings. Refer to Illustrations 9.1 & 9.2.

Hyster, hyster/o means uterus. *Metr, metr/o* also means

uterus
_____.

21.
Hyster/o usually refers to the uterus as a whole organ. Metr/o usu-

uterus
ally refers to the tissues of the _____.

22.
There are exceptions to the rule, but in general hyster/o means the

whole
uterus as a _____ organ. Metr/o refers to the

tissues
_____ of the organ.

23.
Metr/itis means an inflammation of the uterine tissues (linings, mus-

(muscle) tissues of the
cles, etc.). Metr/o/paralysis means paralysis of _____

uterus
_____.

24.
Hyster/o/tomy means incision into the uterus (perhaps to remove a solid tumor). My-, myo- means muscle. What does

muscle tumor of the
hyster/o/my/oma mean? _____

uterus
_____.

25.
Using the word roots hyster, hyster/o, add a suffix from the list and build a new word. Write its meaning in the space provided:

-ectomy   -pathy

hysterectomy
his ter rek′ tō mē
H _____
surgical removal of the
means _____
uterus
_____;

hysteropathy
his ter op′ ō thē
h _____
disease of the uterus
means _____
_____.

26.
Try it again using metr or metr/o. Build a term and then write its meaning:

–scope   –itis
–atrophy (wasting away, diminishing in size)

metroscope
mēt′ rō skōp   M _____
instrument for   means _____
   examining the uterus   _____;

metritis mē trī′ tis   m _____
inflammation of uterine   means _____
   tissues   _____;

metratrophy
mē tra′ trō fē   m _____
                         means _____
uterine tissue atrophy   _____.

27.
Use the word roots metr/, metr/o with the following suffixes to make a new word that fits each of the definitions:

–orrhagia means hemorrhage
–orrhea means flow or discharge

metrorrhagia
mē trō rā′ jē ə   uterine hemorrhage _____;

metrorrhea
mē trō rē′ ə   discharge from the uterus (mucus or pus) _____.

28.
Here are two suffixes that can be confusing:

–orrhexis means rupture (bursting open);
–ocele means hernia or rupture.

The difference between them is the degree of severity of the outcome; the first has a high mortality.

Build a term meaning ruptured uterus (ruptured during labor threatening the mother's life and perhaps the infant's):

hysterorrhexis
his′ ter ō rek′ sis   hyster_____.

Build a term meaning uterine hernia (to be repaired by a surgeon):

hysterocele
his′ ter ō sēl   hyster_____.

endo/myo/metr/itis
en dō mī ō mē trī′ tis

29.
Endo/metr/ium refers to the inside lining of the uterus.
Myo/metr/ium refers to the muscle layer of the uterus.

Build a term meaning inflammation of the inside lining and muscle
layers of the uterus:

_____ / _____ / _____ / _____.
     inside   muscle   uterus   inflammation

hyster, hyster/o
metr, metr/o

30.
Two word roots and their combining forms refer to the uterus.
They are _____ and _____.

hyster/o
metr/o

31.
The term meaning the whole organ is _____. The
term referring to the tissues of the organ is _____.

menstruation
men strū ā′ shun

32.
Now let's look at a uterine function. *Menses, men/o* means monthly
flow of bloody fluid from the uterus. Menstruation is the function
of discharging the menses. Men/o in any word should make you
think of _____.

dis men ō rē′ a
difficult or painful
   menstruation

33.
Men/orrhea means free flow of menses, also known as menstruation.
Dys/men/orrhea means _____.

me nor al′ jē a
painful flow of menses

34.
Men/orrh/algia also means _____
_____.

men ō mē trō rā′ jē ə
excessive bleeding
  (hemorrhage) from
  the uterus during
  menstruation

35.
Try this.

Men/o/metr/orrhagia means _____
_____
_____.

menses
men′ sēs

36.
Menopause is a normal physiological condition of a mature woman.
It's an event that ends a woman's menstrual life. This event marks
the end of her childbearing period. It means the permanent cessation of _____.

children

37.
Menopause means the permanent cessation of the menses. It marks the end of a woman's capability for bearing _____.

38.
Climacteric is a *transitional period* of life sometimes called the change of life. It is a period between ages 45 and 60 when many changes take place in a woman's body. At the end of this transitional period, she no longer experiences menstruation and is no longer capable of bearing a child. The outcome of this transitional period

cessation of menses, or
menopause

is called _____

_____.

39.
During the female climacteric a key physical change takes place. The ovaries permanently and irreversibly atrophy, ending the reproductive period.

This *transitional period* of life is called the climacteric. The outcome of this transition period is the _____, which means _____

complete cessation of
menses

_____.

40.
The *critical period* of life marking the beginning of the end of child-bearing and ending with the onset of menopause is called the

climacteric
klī mak′ ter ik

_____.

41.
Men also experience a decline in sexual activity in their presenile years. This *change of life period* in a man is called the male

climacteric

_____.

42.
Menopause ends the body's reproductive function. What word describes the transitional period of critical changes that ends in menopause? _____.

the climacteric

43.
It's time to review the word combinations you've learned in this section. From the suggested answers, select a term to go with each definition. Write your selection in the space provided.

hysteropathy   mammography
mastodynia   gynecomastia
metrorrhagia   endometritis

gynecomastia   woman's breast (in a male), _____.

hysteropathy   uterine disease, _____.

mastodynia   painful breast, _____.

endometritis   inflammation inside the uterus, _____.

mammography   X ray examination of the breast, _____.

metrorrhagia   uterine hemorrhage, _____.

44.
Here are a few more.

SUGGESTED ANSWERS:

hysterorrhexis   menorrhalgia
amenorrhea   climactric (female)
menopause   metratrophy

menopause   permanent cessation of menses, _____.

amenorrhea   lack of menstruation (temporary), _____.

hysterorrhexis   rupture of uterus (during labor), _____.

climacteric (female) change of life transition period, _____.

menorrhalgia   painful menstruation, _____.

metratrophy   wasting (diminishing in size) of the uterus, _____.

Pregnancy and Childbirth

In this section you'll learn one term at a time. First you'll read a brief paragraph defining the new term. Then you'll answer questions and complete statements about it showing you understand what it means. Feel free to refer back to the paragraph as you work through the frames that follow.

Conception means fertilization. It's an event marked by penetration of the ovum (female egg cell) by a spermatozoon (male germ cell). Conception results in a fertilized ovum. Only a fertilized ovum develops into a human being.

fertilization or
   conception

45.
Penetration of the female egg cell by the male germ cell is known
as _____.

ovum

46.
Another term for female egg cell is _____.

spermatozoon
(sper' ma tō zō' on)

A term meaning male germ cell is _____.

conception

47.
Union of an ovum and a spermatozoon is called _____.

fertilized

A child will develop from an ovum only if the ovum is
_____.

Gestation is the period from conception to childbirth during which
an ovum passes through several stages of development on the way to
becoming a newborn infant. Gestation lasts approximately 9
months, or 280 days from the last menstrual period.

pregnancy

48.
Gestation is another word for the condition known as
_____.

gestation
jes tā' shun

Pregnancy is the condition of a female after conception until the
birth of the baby. Pregnancy is another word for the period of time
called _____.

9
280

49.
Gestation is the process of developing an ovum into a child. It takes
approximately _____ months, or _____ days.

gestation
pregnancy

50.
An ovum develops into a child during a period from conception to
birth. This process is called _____ and the condition is called _____.

gestation

51.
During pregnancy an ovum passes through many developmental
stages or phases. Taken together, these phases make up the nine-
month period called _____.

The earliest gestational phase begins with a fertilized female egg
cell. In just two weeks, the ovum divides into two cells, and each
cell continues halving until it has become a complex mass of cells.

This mass of cells is now called an *embryo*. It's a living organism ready to continue its development into the next phase.

52.
The indispensable event that initiates a pregnancy is

conception

_____.

ovum
ō′ vum
two

53.
After conception, the earliest phase of development begins with a fertilized _____ and lasts _____ weeks.

54.
The first two weeks of gestation produce a complex living organism called a/an _____.

embryo
em′ brē ō

The *embryo* begins a second stage of gestation in the third week, which lasts six weeks. In the third week, the embryo begins to acquire structure (head, arms, legs, and a tail), and over the next few weeks it begins forming principal internal organs and body systems. By the end of the eighth week of gestation the embryo looks somewhat like a human and is called a *fetus*.

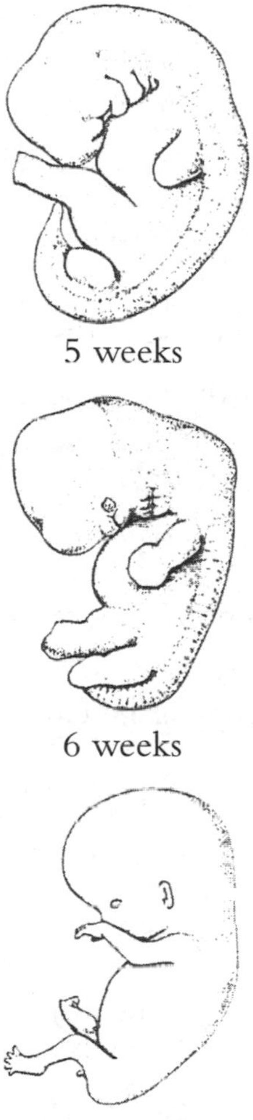

5 weeks

55.
The second stage of gestation begins with a two-week-old ovum, which is now called an

embryo

_____.

6 weeks

56.
The embryo begins its second stage of development in the _____ week of gestation and continues through the _____ week of a new pregnancy. At the beginning of the ninth week, it is called a _____.

third

eighth

fetus

8 weeks

Figure 9.315

57.
During this second gestational phase the embryo begins forming
organs arms and legs and principal internal _____.

human being 58.
fetus By the beginning of the ninth week, the embryo begins to resemble
fē′ tus a _____ and is called a _____.

59.
A *fetus* begins the last phase of gestation. A fetus is a live offspring
while it is in the mother (in utero). It continues developing during
the remainder of the gestational period. The fetal stage lasts from
the beginning of the third month of gestation to childbirth. A fetus
sufficiently developed to sustain life outside the uterus is called a
viable fetus.

In the last gestational phase, the fetus in utero develops into a
viable fetus _____.

at three months of When does this phase begin? _____
  pregnancy _____.

seven more months How long does it last? _____.

childbirth What is the terminating event? _____.

60.
Here's a quick review.

• Penetration of an ovum by a spermatozoon is called
conception _____.

• A nine-month period during which a fertilized ovum becomes a
pregnancy or gestation child is called _____.

• In the first two weeks of pregnancy an ovum becomes a complex
embryo organism called an _____.

• From the third week to the beginning of the ninth week of
pregnancy an embryo develops rudimentary appendages and
organs internal _____.

a human being • After only two months' gestation, the embryo begins to resemble
fetus _____ and is called a _____.

• A fetus developing in utero for the next seven months becomes a
human being or child _____.

childbirth • Gestation ends with _____.

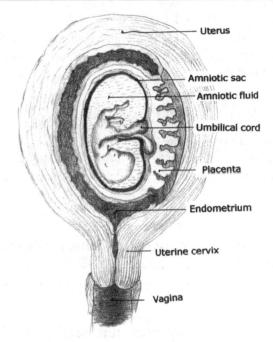

Figure 9.4.   Fetus in Utero, Beginning 9th Week.

uterus (hyster/o, metr/o)
amniotic sac (amni/o, amniot/o)
amniotic fluid (liquor amnii)

61.
Here are a few medical terms referring to some structures and conditions relating to pregnancy. *Amnion, amni/o, amniot/o* refer to a thin transparent sac containing the fetus and the fluid surrounding the fetus. This sac grows rapidly as the fetus inside develops. The amniotic fluid protects the fetus from injury and helps maintain an even temperature.

amniotic fluid
am nē ot′ ik flū′ id

Within the amniotic sac the fetus is protected from injury and changes in temperature by the *liquor amnii*, or in other words,

_____.

62.

amniotic

Amniot/itis means inflammation of the amnion. Build a word that means pertaining to the sac that envelops the fetus: _____.

am′ nē ō sen tē′ sis
puncturing the amniotic
   sac and withdrawing
   some fluid

63.
Centesis is the suffix meaning to puncture a cavity and remove fluid. Explain the meaning of amni/o/centesis: _____

_____.

am′ nē ō tōm
usually an ultrasound
  graphic study of
  the amnion (and its
  contents)

64.
Amni/o/tome is an instrument for cutting (puncturing) the amnion. What does amni/ography mean? _____
_____
_____.

ol′ i gō hī dram′ nē os
scanty amount of
  amniotic fluid in
  the sac

65.
Olig-, oligo- is a prefix meaning little, small, scanty. Olig/uria means scanty urination. What does oligo/hydr/amnios mean? _____
_____
_____.

excessive amount of
  amniotic fluid in the
  sac

66.
What do you think polyhydramnios means?
_____
_____.

amniotic sac or amnion

67.
What structure envelops the fetus and contains the fluid protecting the fetus? _____.

68.
Placenta is a structure made up of a network of blood vessels (arteries and veins). The placenta makes an intimate bond with the inside lining of the uterus (endometrium), and attaches to the fetus by the umbilical cord. The fetus absorbs oxygen and nutrients from its mother through the placenta. It excretes carbon dioxide and other wastes through this same vascular structure. The placenta begins to form about the eighth day of gestation, and by the end of the pregnancy weighs about one-sixth the weight of the infant. After the birth of the child, the uterus expels the placenta, now called the *afterbirth*.

The fetus in utero absorbs oxygen and nutrients and excretes carbon dioxide and wastes through a vascular structure called the

placenta

_____.

1 pound
1 ounce

69.
The placenta weighs one-sixth of the weight of the infant. If the baby's birth weight is 6 pounds, 6 ounces, what would you expect the placenta to weigh at the end of pregnancy? _____ pound _____ ounce.

en dō mē′ trē um
the inside lining of the
    uterus

70.
The placenta forms and grows on the endometrium and makes an intimate bond with it. What is the endometrium? _____
_____.

71.
While in utero the fetus grows by getting its nourishment through

placenta
umbilical cord

the _____. The fetus is attached to the placenta by the _____.

afterbirth

72.
The placenta is expelled after the baby is born. The placenta is also called _____.

pregnant (a current
    condition)

73.
Gravida, gravid refers to a pregnant woman; being heavy with child. Gravidism is the condition of being _____.

prī′ ma grav′ i da
a woman who *is*
    pregnant with her
    first child

74.
Primi- means first; *secundi-* means second. Primigravida refers to

_____

_____.

What do you think gravida II means?

a woman in her second
    pregnancy

_____

_____.

secundigravida
sē kun′ da grav′ i da

Build a compound medical term meaning a woman in her second pregnancy: _____.

75.
Here's a quick review. From the suggested answers, select a term to go with each definition. Write your selection in the space provided.

SUGGESTED ANSWERS:
oligohydramnios   primigravida
amniocentesis   secundigravida
amniotic fluid   placenta

secundigravida

a woman in her second pregnancy, _____.

primigravida

a pregnant woman, first time, _____.

oligohydramnios

scanty fluid in the amnion, _____.

placenta	fetus in utero absorbs nutrients and excretes waste through it, _____.
amniotic fluid	*liquor amnii,* _____.
amniocentesis	puncture of the amnion and removal of fluid, _____.

Labor and Delivery

Parturition is more commonly known as *labor.* Parturition is the process by which a baby is born and the placenta expelled from the uterus. This labor, or parturition, has three stages. The first stage is the stage of *dilation.* It is characterized by contractions of the uterine muscle and dilation of the birth canal and cervix—to let the baby out. The second stage is *expulsion.* The baby is born! In the third stage the placenta is expelled. This is the *afterbirth* stage. The average duration of labor is about 13 hours in primagravida women (12 hours in dilation stage, 1 hour in expulsion stage, and a few minutes for the afterbirth). Labor is about 8 hours long in subsequent pregnancies.

76.
At term, when gestation is completed, a spontaneous physiological process begins. It has three stages: dilation, expulsion, and afterbirth. This process is called _____ OR _____.

parturition
labor

77.
In the first stage of labor, the uterus contracts rhythmically for 8 to 12 hours. The cervix stretches and opens until it is fully dilated so the baby may pass through the birth canal. This first stage is called the _____ stage.

dilation
dī lā′ shun

78.
The second stage of labor involves expulsion. The infant passes through the birth canal and is _____.

expelled, born

79.
Expulsion of the placenta follows the birth of the child. The expelled placenta is more commonly known as the _____.

afterbirth

80.
What happens during the expulsion stage, or the second stage of labor? _____.

a child is born
   (expelled)

a few minutes

the placenta is expelled

81.
How long is the third stage of labor? _____.

What happens in the afterbirth stage of labor? _____

_____.

---

the cervix (neck of the
uterus) completely
dilates (opens)

82.
After 8 to 12 hours of uterine contractions during the first stage of labor, what has happened?

_____ _____

_____.

---

par tyer ish' un
labor

83.
Parturition is another word for childbirth. What other term you just learned also means the process of being born? _____.

84.
Antepartum refers to the entire gestational period before labor begins.

pertaining to after labor
is completed

What does postpartum mean? _____

_____.

---

pertaining to the recent
period around
childbirth

85.
Neo means new or recent. *Natus* is a Latin term for birth. What does neonatal mean? _____

_____.

---

pertaining to medical
care and supervision
of a pregnant woman
before childbirth

86.
What do you think prenatal care means? _____

_____

_____.

87.
Review the terms you just learned before moving on. Select the term that best fits each brief definition. Use the suggestions if you need help.

labor   parturition
prenatal care   afterbirth
dilation   expulsion

prenatal care
prē nā' tal kair

medical supervision of a pregnant woman, _____

_____.

labor or parturition

the process of giving birth, _____ _____.

parturition or labor	the act of childbirth, _____.
dilation	first stage of labor, _____.
expulsion	second stage of labor, _____.
afterbirth	third stage of labor, _____.

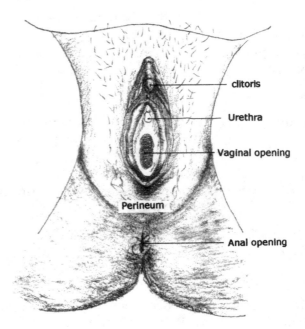

Figure 9.5.   Female Pudenda.

urethra (urethr/o)   perineum
vagina (vagin/o)   anus (an/o)

88.
Pudendum, pudenda (plural) means the external genitals (sex organs) of a female. These parts are easily observed without manual examination.

Take a look at Illustration 9.5 above.

pudendal
pyoo den′ dl

Build a term meaning pertaining to the female's external genitals: _____.

89.
Perineum refers to the structures that make up the pelvic outlet and comprise the pelvic floor. It is the region between the lip at the vaginal opening and anus in a female or between the scrotum

anus
ā′ nus

and _____ in a male.

perineum
per i nē′ um

90.
A baby coming through the birth canal during parturition can over-stretch the vagina and the pelvic outlet. A tear (laceration) may occur in the tissues around the pelvic outlet. This pelvic floor structure is called the _____.

91.
Episiotomy is an incision of the perineum. During the second stage of labor, just before the baby is born, the obstetrician may incise the perineum to avoid a more damaging laceration of the surrounding tissues.

Episiotomy controls damage to the tissues of the vagina and

perineum

_____.

episiotomy
e pēz ē ot′ ō mē

92.
An incision into the perineum is called _____.

suturing repair,
reconstruction of
the tissues after an
episiotomy

93.
What does episiorrhaphy mean? _____

_____

_____.

94.
Here's a term often confused with perineum. *Peritoneum* is a tough membrane covering the viscera (organs in the belly) and lining the abdominal cavity. It clings to the viscera as plastic wrap clings to whatever it covers.

peritoneum
per i tō nē′ um

per i tō nī′ tis
inflammation of the
peritoneum

The membrane that coats the viscera and lines the abdominal cavity is the _____.
                perineum/peritoneum

What is peritonitis? _____

_____.

95.
Select one of the terms that best fits the brief definition. Write it in the space provided.

peritoneum   episiotomy
pudenda   perineum

pudenda

external female genitals, _____.

perineum

the region of the external female genitals between the vaginal lip and anus, _____.

peritoneum	a membrane coating the viscera and lining the abdominal cavity, _____.
episiotomy	incision of the perineum to limit injury of the pelvic outlet during childbirth, _____.

96.
Involution is a *process* the body goes through that reduces the uterus to its normal nonpregnant size and condition following childbirth.

involution	The process that returns an enlarged uterus to its normal size after the baby is born is called _____.

97.
Puerperium is a *period of time* following the third stage of labor when involution takes place. Involution lasts approximately six weeks.

poo er pēr′ ē um expelled	Puerperium begins after the fetus and the placenta have been _____.

98.
Puerperium lasts until the uterus returns to its size and condition before pregnancy began. This period of time is approximately

six	_____ weeks.

99.
After fulfilling its function, the uterus goes through a process of returning to its earlier nonpregnant condition. This process is called

involution	_____.

100.

puerperium poo er pēr′ ē um	Involution takes place during a six-week period after childbirth. This time period is called the _____.

101.

of or pertaining to the period after childbirth when involution takes place	Explain the meaning of the term puerperal. _____ _____ _____.

102.
Sepsis means the presence of pathogenic organisms or bacteria that cause serious infections. Years ago, prior to effective antibiotic therapy, the greatest single cause of death following childbirth was called *childbed fever.*

puerperal (sepsis)	Another description of this condition is _____ sepsis.
	<div align="right">(pertaining to the time when involution takes place)</div>

inflammation of the
  peritoneum during
  puerperium

103.
What is puerperal peritonitis? _____
_____.

the process by which
  the uterus returns
  to its earlier
  nonpregnant state
  after childbirth

104.
Involution takes place during puerperium. What does involution
mean? _____
_____
_____.

nulli/para
nullipara
nu lip′ ə ra

105.
Nulli- is a prefix meaning none. *Para* means to bear a child. Build a
term that refers to a woman who has never borne a child:
_____ / _____.

prīm ip′ ə ra
a woman who has
  given birth to one
  viable child (an event
  in the past)

106.
A woman who has delivered more than one living child is described
as *multipara*. What does *primipara* mean? _____
_____
_____.

she has given birth to
  two viable children

107.
What does an obstetrician mean when he writes in the patient's
chart that she is para-2? _____
_____.

108.
Using the word root *para* and *nulli-*, *multi-*, or *primi-*, build a word
for each of the following abbreviations.

primipara
nullipara
multipara
mul tip′ ə ra

para-1, _____.
para-0, _____.
para-4, _____.

109.
It's a good time to review what you just covered. Select a term
from the suggestions and complete each brief definition.

nullipara   parturition
primigravida   antepartum
involution   puerperium

involution

the process taking place after childbirth that reduces the uterus to
normal size and condition, _____.

puerperium	the six-week period after childbirth when involution takes place, _____.
antepartum	the period in a pregnancy occurring before labor, _____.
nullipara	a woman who has never given birth to a viable child, _____.
primigravida	a woman who is pregnant for the first time ever, _____.
parturition	another term for labor, _____.

110.
Here are some terms you may find very interesting. Look them up in your medical dictionary. You'll be surprised at how much you have learned.

acquired	congenital
anomaly	eclampsia
placenta abruptio	placenta previa

111.
Here are 50 new words you worked with in this unit. When you pronounce each term be sure to think about what it means. Then take the Unit 9 Self-Test.

amenorrhea (ä men ō rē′ a)
amniocentesis (am′ nē ō sen tē′ sis)
amnion (am′ nē on)
amniotic fluid (am nē ôt ik floo′ id)
climacteric (klī mak′ ter ik)
conception (kon sep′ shun)
dysmenorrhea (dis men ōr ē′ ə)
embryo
endometrium
  (en′ dō mē′ trē um)
episiotomy (e pēz ē ot′ ō mē)
fetus
gestation (jes tā′ shun)
gynecomastia (gī′ ne kō mas′ tē ə)
gynoplasty (jin′ ō plas tē)
hysterocele (his′ ter ō sēl)
hysteromyoma
  (his′ ter ō mī ō′ mä)

hysterorrhexis
  (his′ ter ō rek′ sis)
involution (in vō loo′ shun)
labor
mammalgia (ma mal′ jē ə)
mammary (mam′ ə rē)
mammopexy (mam′ ō pek sē)
mastodynia (mas tō din′ ē ə)
mastoncus (mas tong′ kus)
mastopathy (mas top′ ə thē)
mastoptosis (mas top tō′ sis)
menometrorrhagia
  (men′ ō mētrō rā′ jē ə)
menopause (men′ ō pawz)
menorrhalgia (men ō ral′ jē ə)
menses (men′ sēz)
menstruation
  (men strū ā′ shun)

metratrophy (mē tra′ trō fē)

metrorrhagia (mē trō ra′ jē ə)

multipara (mul tip′ ə ra)

myometritis (mī′ ō mē trī′ tis)

neonatal (nē ō nā′ tal)

nullipara (nu lip′ ə ra)

oligohydramnios
(ol′ ē gō hī dram′ nē ōs)

ovum (ō′ vum)

parturition (pär tyo͞or ish′ un)

perineum (per i nē′ um)

peritoneum (per i tō nē′ um)

placenta

polyhydramnios
(pä lē hī dram′ nē ōs)

postpartum

primigravida
(prī′ ma grav′ i da)

pudenda (pyo͞o den′ də)

puerperal sepsis
(po͞o er′ per al sep sis)

puerperium
(po͞o er pēr′ ē um)

spermatozoon
(sper′ ma tō zō′ on)

Unit 9 Self-Test

Part 1

From the right, select the correct meaning for each of the following medical terms.

_____	1. Primigravida	a. X ray study of the breast
_____	2. Pudenda	b. Temporary lack of menstruation
_____	3. Hysteropathy	c. Pelvic floor, region from vaginal lip to anus
_____	4. Mammary	
_____	5. Mastrodynia	d. Process returning uterus to non-pregnant state
_____	6. Amniotic	e. Incision of vagina and pelvic outlet
_____	7. Episiotomy	f. Female external genitals
_____	8. Endometritis	g. Pregnant woman, first time
_____	9. Involution	h. Period after childbirth, when involution takes place
_____	10. Metratrophy	
_____	11. Perineum	i. Pertaining to sac holding the fetus and fluid
_____	12. Amenorrhea	j. Rupture of uterus (during labor)
_____	13. Puerperium	k. Pertaining to the breast
_____	14. Hysterorrhexis	l. Uterine atrophy (wasting)
_____	15. Mammography	m. Inflammation of uterine inside lining
		n. Painful breasts
		o. Uterine disease

Part 2

Write the medical term for each of the following brief definitions.

1. Surgical fixation of pendulous breasts   _____

2. Membrane covering abdominal viscera (organs)   _____

3. Painful breasts   _____

4. Change of life period   Female _____

5. Organism in utero resembling a human   _____

6. Organ that nourishes fetus in utero   _____

7. Surgical removal of the breast   _____

8. Another term for pregnancy   _____

9. Pertaining to a recently born child   _____

10. Woman pregnant with her first child   _____

11. Pendulous breast   _____

12. Fertilization of an ovum   _____

13. Labor and delivery of term pregnancy   _____

14. Pertaining to before the onset of labor   _____

15. After childbirth when involution takes place   P _____

ANSWERS

Part 1	Part 2
1. g	1. Mammopexy
2. f	2. Peritoneum
3. o	3. Mastodynia, mammalgia
4. k	4. Female climacteric
5. n	5. Fetus
6. i	6. Placenta
7. e	7. Mastectomy
8. m	8. Gestation
9. d	9. Neonatal

10. l   10. Primipara
11. c   11. Mastoptosis
12. b   12. Conception
13. h   13. Parturition
14. j   14. Antepartum
15. a   15. Puerperium

10 The Eye and the Respiratory Tract

Unit 10 is divided into two sections. In the first section you'll work with new terms relating to the eye. You will use some new word roots and combining forms and put them together with many suffixes you are already familiar with. The second section covers new terms relating to the respiratory tract. Review the Mini-Glossary below.

Mini-Glossary

The Eye

blephar/o (*eyelid*)

core, core/o (*pupil*)

corne/o, kerat/o (*cornea*)

cycl/o (*ciliary body*)

dipl/o (*paired, double*)

ir, irid/o (*iris*)

lacrim/o (*tear*)

ophthalm/o (*eye*)

retin/o (*retina*)

scler/o (*sclera*)

The Respiratory Tract

bronch/i (*bronch/o, bronchus*)

laryng/o (*voice box*)

ment/o (*chin*)

nas/o (*nose*)

pharyng/o (*throat*)

pleur/o (*covering of the lung*)

pneum/o (*air, breathe*)

pneumon/o (*lung*)

thorac/o (*thorax*)

trache/o (*windpipe*)

Don't forget to complete the Review Sheet for Unit 9 before beginning Unit 10. Keep up the good work!

1.

Let's refresh your memory. You'll find it helpful to review suffixes you already studied and will use again in the first section. Write the meaning of each of the following. Do your best without looking at the answers.

"charley horse," twitching	–spasm _____
suturing, repair	–orrhaphy _____
inflammation of	–itis _____
a diseased condition	–pathy _____
instrument that cuts	–tome _____
dilation, stretching	–ectasia _____
resembling, like	–oid _____
to fix, fixation (into normal place)	–pexy _____
pertaining to out of normal place	–ectopic _____
hernia, herniation	–cele _____
drooping, prolapse	–ptosis _____
measuring, measuring instrument	metr-, –meter _____
instrument for examining, looking inside of	–scope, –scopy _____
treatment, treating a condition	–therapy _____
surgery to restore or make new	–plasty _____

2.

Now, let's try it the other way. Write the suffix that satisfies the definition given in the table below. Then go back to the first frame and check your answers. You may want to use this table to help you complete the next few frames.

Definition	Suffix
to measure, instrument for measuring	
treatment for a condition	
inflammation of	
dilation, stretch	
drooping, prolapse	
examine, instrument to look inside	
surgery to restore, make new	
resembling, like	
"charley horse," twitching	
a diseased condition	
surgically fix into normal place	
suture, repair after trauma	
instrument for cutting	
pertaining to out of normal place	
hernia, rupture	

The Eye

of, pertaining to, or
   relating to the eye

opthalm-
ophthalm/o

3.

Here are some new terms. Ophthalmology is the medical specialty concerned with the eye, and its diseases. Ophthalm/o/malacia means an abnormal softening of the eyeball.
What is the word root? _____ Write the combining form: _____.

4.

Ophthalm, ophthalm/o are the word root and combining form for terms difficult to spell and pronounce. But if you pronounce the words correctly, the spelling will be easier. For example, oph/thal/mo is pronounced of thal′ mō. The oph is pronounced as _____. In the word root ophthalm-, ph comes before th, as in the alphabet (p before t). Oph thal mō is pronounced _____.

of

of thal′ mō

Pronounce it.

5.

Here's a chance to practice your spelling and pronunciation. Use the combining form ophthalm/o and add each of these suffixes to build new words.

-cele   hernia, herniation
-meter   instrument for measuring
-plegia   paralysis

Build a term and then pronounce it carefully:

ophthalmocele
of thal′ mō sēl

herniation of the eye (abnormal protrusion), _____;

ophthalmometer
of′ thal mom′ e ter

instrument for measuring the eye, _____;

ophthalmoplegia
of thal′ mo plē′ gē a

paralysis of the eye (eye muscle), _____.

6.

ophthalmologist
of thal mol′ ō jist

The physician who practices the medical specialty concerned with diseases of the eye is an _____.

7.

ophthalmoscope
of thal′ mō skōp

The instrument used for examining the interior of the eyeball through the pupil is an _____.

8.

double vision

Dipl/o means double or paired. -*Opia* is a suffix meaning vision. What does dipl/opia mean? _____.

9.

diplopia
di plō′ pē a

Whenever a pair of eyes fail to record a singular image in the brain, a double image occurs. The medical term for double vision is _____.

10.

double (or paired)
    bacteria
bluish vision

Write a brief meaning for each of the following.
dipl/o/bacteria, _____
_____;
cyan/opia; _____.

11.

blef a rop′ tō sis
blephar-
blephar/o

Blephar/optosis means prolapse (drooping) of an eyelid. The word root for eyelid is _____. The combining form is _____.

blef ar e dē′ ma
blephar<u>edema</u>

12.
Blephar/edema means excess fluid in the tissues of the eyelid.
Underline the part of the term meaning swelling due to fluid in the tissues: blephar<u>edema</u>.

blepharedema

13.
The condition of swollen eyelids due to excess fluid in the eyelids is

_____.

14.
Define each of the following terms:

blef′ ar ō spazm
twitching of the eyelid

blepharospasm means _____

_____.

blef ar ōr′ a fē
suturing of the eyelid

blepharorrhaphy means _____

_____.

blef ar ī′ tis
blepharitis

15.
Build a word that means inflammation of the eyelid,

_____.

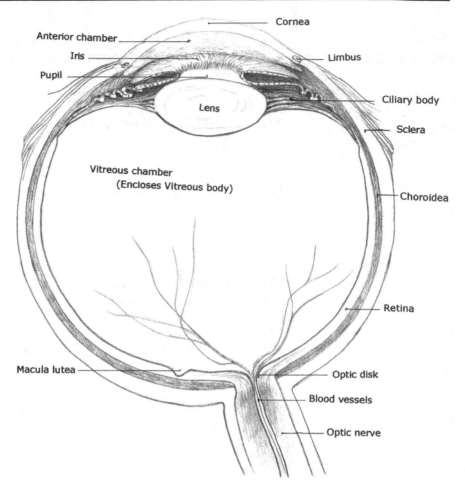

Figure 10.1   The Eye.

Sight is the most dominant of the human senses. Over 70% of the body's receptors are the specialized photosensitive cells of the eyes. It has been estimated that a third of all the fibers bringing impulses to the central nervous system come from the eye.

The human eye is somewhat like a camera that captures light and focuses it on a light-sensitive area. The wall of the eyeball consists of three coats or layers of tissue. The first layer is the fibrous, rubber-like protective coat called the *sclera,* known as the "white of the eye." The sclera gives the eyeball its shape, and can be seen around most of the eyeball's surface. A continuation of the sclera and the most anterior segment of this fibrous coat is the cornea. The *cornea* is a transparent structure that bulges and has no blood vessels. It plays a big role in focusing light rays on the retina of the eye. The area called the *limbus* is where the cornea meets the sclera.

The middle layer of the eyeball is the vascular layer called the *choroidea*. It lies between the retinal and the scleral layers. The choroidea contains many blood vessels and includes the iris and the ciliary body. The iris, or the colored part of the eye seen through the cornea, is a fibromuscular body that circumscribes the hole (pupil) in front of the lens. Action of the iris increases and decreases the size of the pupil. Another portion of the choroidea is the ciliary body. This structure is continuous with the iris and contains the ciliary muscle, which controls eye movement. The lens is a tightly packed and encapsulated bunch of special fibers. Along with the cornea, it shares responsibility for bringing images into focus on the retina.

The fluid-filled space between the iris and the cornea is the *anterior chamber.* It contains a fluid material called aqueous humor which services the cells within its environment. A large cavity posterior to the lens is known as the *vitreous chamber.* This cavity contains a clear, gelatinous mass known as the vitreous body. The vitreous body maintains the shape of the eye and gives support to the retina.

The *retina* is the the innermost coat of the eye, the neural layer. It lines a bit more than the posterior half of the globe. The retina is a complexly composed network of interlacing layers of blood vessels and photoreceptor cells that come together at the *optic disk.* This is actually a blind spot since there are no photoreceptors here. The optic disk penetrates the wall of the eye and forms the optic nerve which carries impulses to the brain.

When light enters the eye, it passes through the cornea, pupil, and lens, and focuses an image on the retina. At about the center of the retina there is a clearly depressed region with a dense accumulation of photoreceptor cells. This area of the retina providing the sharpest vision is called the *macula lutea.* At the center of macula is the *fovea centralis.* This site represents the center of the greatest visual acuity (clarity of form and color) under lighted conditions.

I hope you enjoyed your tour of the anatomy of the eye.

cornea (kerat/o)	sclera (skler/o)
iris (ir, irid, irid/o)	pupil (cor, core/o)
retina (retin/o)	ciliary body (cycl/o)

16.
Use Illustration 10.1, The Eye, and the accompanying description. The cornea is the transparent tissue covering the anterior sixth of the eye. *Kerat, kerat/o* form words referring to the cornea. Write the meaning of each of the following:

kor nē al
pertaining to the
  cornea

corneal _____ ;

ker a top′ a thē
disease of the cornea

kerat/o/pathy _____ .

17.

keratoplasty
ker′ a tō plas tē

Using the combining form kerat/o, build a term meaning plastic repair of the cornea: _____ .

18.

kerat, kerat/o

The cornea is one-sixth of the outer coat of the eyeball. It is the transparent tissue covering the front of the eyeball. The word root and combining form meaning cornea are _____ .

19.

cornea

Scler/o refers to the white of the eye. The sclera is the hard fibrous coat forming the outer envelope of the eye. It covers five-sixths of the eyeball. The other anterior sixth is occupied by the _____ .

20.
Corneoscleral means pertaining to an area where the cornea meets the sclera. Write the meaning for each of the following:

skler′ al
pertaining to the sclera

scleral _____
_____ ;

skler′ ō tōm
instrument for cutting
  the sclera

sclerotome _____
_____ .

21.

sclerectomy
skle rek′ tō mē

Sclerectasia means bulging (stretching) of the white of the eye. Build a term meaning excision of a portion of the sclera:
_____ .

ī′ ris
ir′ i dō kor′ nē al
pertaining to the area
    where the iris and
    cornea meet

22.
Iris means rainbow. The iris is a diaphragm perforated in the center (the pupil). The word roots referring to the donut-shaped color in the eye are *ir, irid,* and *irid/o.* What do you think iridocorneal means? _____

_____

ir′ id ō sēl
hernia of the iris

Iridocele means _____

_____

ir/itus
iritis
ī rī′ tis

23.
One of the word roots for the iris is ir. It has very limited use, but it's always used to express inflammation.

Using the word root ir build a word meaning inflammation of the iris: _____ / _____.

i ri dal′ jē ə
pain in the iris

24.
Irid/o is the combining form used to refer to the iris in almost all other words. Iridalgia means _____.

iridectomy
i ri dek′ tō mē

25.
Build a term meaning excision of part of the iris:

_____.

26.
Write what each of the following word roots or combining forms means.

cornea
vision, sight
iris
sclera
eye
eyelid
iris

kerat/o, _____.
opia, _____.
irid/o, _____.
scler/o, _____.
ophthalm/o, _____.
blephar/o, _____.
ir, _____.

retinal
ret′ i n'l
retinitis
ret i nī′ tis
retinoid
ret′ i noyd

27.
Retin/o refers to the complex membrane lining the inside back surface of the eye. It receives the visual light rays, which the brain interprets and gives meaning. Build a word meaning

pertaining to the retina, _____;

inflammation of the retina, _____;

resembling the retina, _____.

retinoscope or
   ophthalmoscope
ret′ i nō skōp

28.
Retinopexy means affixing (or adhering) the retina to the wall of the eyeball for correcting retinal detachment. What would you call an instrument for examining the retina to look for retinopathy?

_____.

ret i nop′ a thē
disease of the retina

29.
What does retinopathy mean? _____

_____.

(eye), iris

30.
The pupil is the circular opening in the center of the iris through which the light rays enter the eye. It is the core or center of the eye. *Cor, core/o* refer to the pupil in the center of the _____.

31.
An ophthalmologist may use drops in the eye to dilate the pupil before an examination.

Analyze the term cor/ectasia.

pupil

Cor- is the root meaning _____;

dilation

ectasia means _____.

kōr ek tō′ pē a
a misplaced pupil

What does cor/ectopia mean? _____

_____.

kōr ē om′ e trē
measuring the size of a
   pupil

32.
Coreoplasty is a surgical procedure for correcting a deformed pupil.

Write a term meaning to measure the size of a pupil. _____

_____.

sī klō pa ral′ i sis
paralysis of the ciliary
   body

33.
Take another look at Illustration 10.1, The Eye. The ciliary body controls movement of the eye. The word root for ciliary body is *cycl/o*. It means circle or surrounding.

What does cyclo/paralysis mean? _____

_____.

sī klō krī′ ō ther′ a pē
cyclo<u>cryo</u>therapy

34.
Cyclocryotherapy means freezing of the ciliary body in the treatment of glaucoma. Underline the part of the term referring to freezing: cyclocryotherapy.

sī klō ker a tī′ tis
inflammation of the
    cornea and the
    ciliary body

35.
Use Illustration 10.1 for help. Cyclitis means inflammation of the ciliary body. What is the meaning of cyclokeratitis? _____
_____
_____.

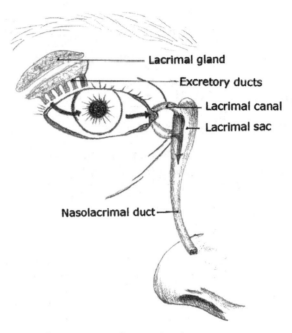

Figure 10.2 The Lacrimal apparatus.

    The human lacrimal apparatus is responsible for producing tears and delivering them to the eye. When an excess is produced, the tears flow into the nasal cavities.

    The lacrimal apparatus begins with the *lacrimal gland* seen under the upper lateral eyebrow and extending inward toward the midline. Blinking stimulates the lacrimal gland to secrete lacrimal fluid (tears) that washes the eye. It also contains substances that destroy the cell walls of bacteria, and it moistens the surface of the eye. The fluid passes through a series of excretory ducts and enters a fold of tissue under the upper eyelid. The eyelid then distributes the tears across the eyeball. Excess fluid flows to the medial corner of the eye passing through a tiny opening and entering the *lacrimal canal*. The upper and lower lacrimal canals drain into the *lacrimal sac*. Excess tears move from the lacrimal sac into the *nasolacrimal duct* and pass through an opening into the nose. This is the reason one sniffles when crying.

36.
Look again at the illustration. The lacrimal apparatus consists of the gland, the sac, and the duct. The purpose of the lacrimal apparatus is to keep the surface of the eye moist and protected. What do you think lacrimal means? _____.

lak′ ri mal
relating to tears

37.
The gland that secretes tears is the _____ gland.

lacrimal

The sac that collects the tears is the _____ sac.

lacrimal

What is the structure that empties the tears into the nasal cavity? _____ _____.

nasolacrimal duct

38.
Tears keep the surface of the eye moistened. Tears are continually being formed and removed. When tears form more quickly than they can be removed by the lacrimal apparatus, we say the person is _____.

crying

39.
How about a review? Complete each of the following brief definitions. Use the suggested answers to help you.

SUGGESTED ANSWERS:

iritis	cycloplegia
lacrimal	diplopia
cyclocryotherapy	sclerotome
retinoscopy	ophthalmic
coreometry	keratitis
iridocele	keratoplasty

coreometry   measurement of pupil size, _____.
iridocele   herniation of the iris, _____.
ophthalmic   pertaining to the eye, _____.
retinoscopy   examination of the retina, _____.
iritis   inflammation of the iris, _____.
sclerotome   instrument for cutting the sclera, _____.
lacrimal   relating to tears, _____.
keratoplasty   surgical reconstruction of the cornea, _____.
cycloplegia   paralytic ciliary body, _____.
keratitis   inflammation of the cornea, _____.
diplopia   double vision, _____.
cyclocryotherapy treatment (of glaucoma) freezing the ciliary body,

_____.

40.

Try these now. Write the meaning of each of the following word roots:

retina	retin/o, _____.
pupil	cor/o, core/o, _____.
ciliary body	cycl/o, _____.
eyelid	blephar/o, _____.
cornea	kerat/o (corne/o), _____.
eye	ophthalm/o, _____.
sight, vision	opia, _____.
iris	irid/o, _____.

The Respiratory Tract

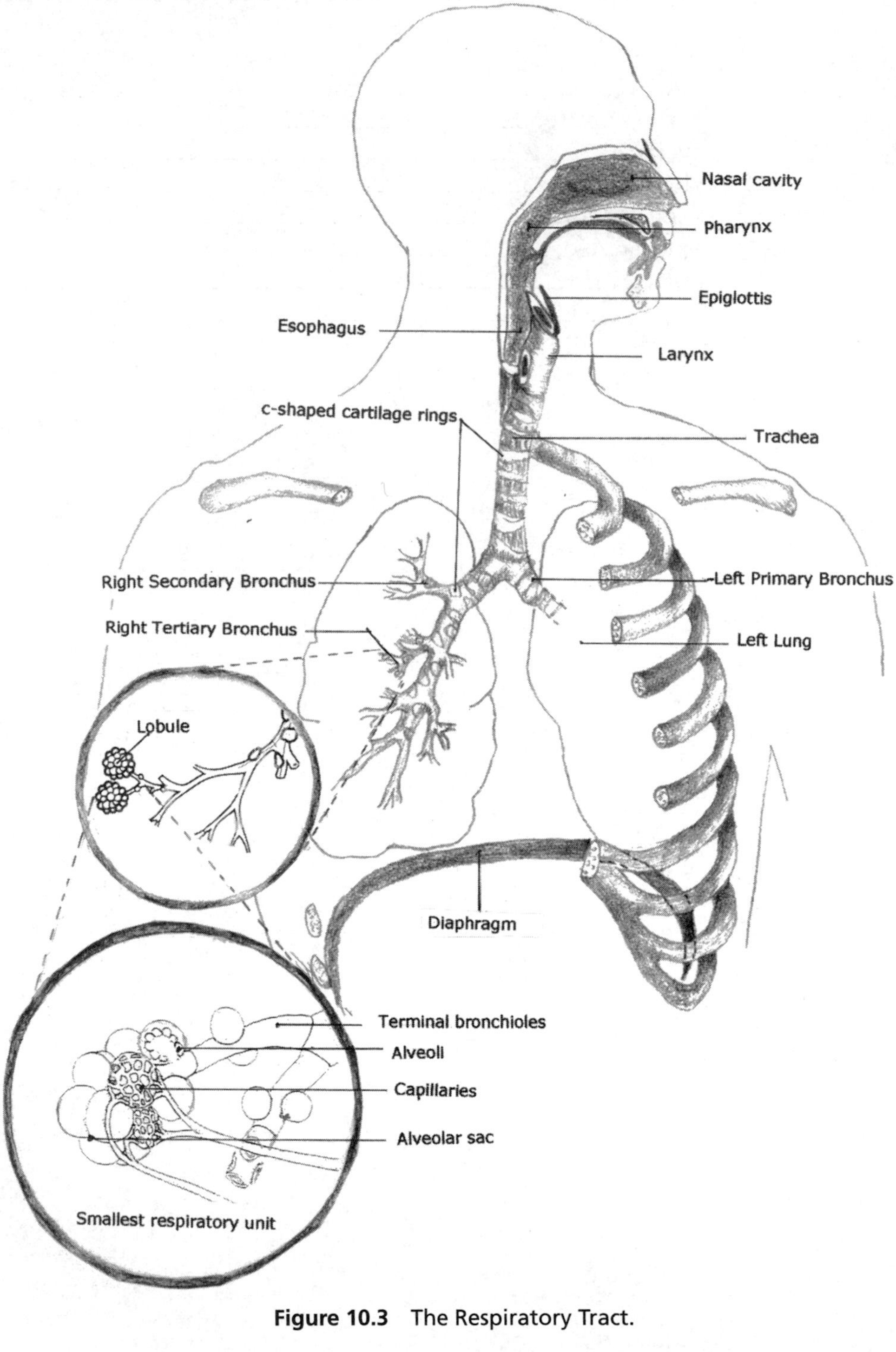

Nasal cavity

Pharynx

Epiglottis

Esophagus

Larynx

c-shaped cartilage rings

Trachea

Right Secondary Bronchus

Left Primary Bronchus

Right Tertiary Bronchus

Left Lung

Lobule

Diaphragm

Terminal bronchioles

Alveoli

Capillaries

Alveolar sac

Smallest respiratory unit

Figure 10.3   The Respiratory Tract.

The respiratory system consists of passageways that receive incoming air and carry it to the *lungs* for exchange of oxygen and carbon dioxide gases. The lungs are the main organs of gas exchange in the body. They are soft, spongy organs enveloped in a tough, wet and slippery transparent membrane called the *pleura*. The lungs are protected by the bony cage of the thorax. Most of the rest of the skeleton of the respiratory tract is cartilaginous, right down to the smallest air passageway. The dome–shaped muscular *diaphragm* provides most of the force necessary for inspiration and expiration of air. One quarter of the force is generated by the intercostal muscles moving the ribs. When the diaphragm contracts and flattens in its space, air enters the lungs. When it relaxes, air is expelled from the lungs.

Air enters the respiratory tract through the oral and nasal cavities. The *nasal cavity* houses the olfactory sense organ used in the sense of smell. The *pharynx* is an open area continuous with the nasal cavity, and its lower end opens to the *esophagus* and *larynx*. These upper passageways warm, moisten and purify the air on its way to the lower respiratory tract.

The *larynx* is an enlarged section of the upper respiratory tract at the top of the trachea. The opening to the larynx is guarded by a leaf–like flap of cartilage called the *epiglottis*. This structure prevents food from entering the respiratory passageway and directs it to the esophagus. Beneath the epiglottis is the opening to the larynx called the *glottis*. The larynx houses the vocal cords, an important component of the larynx used in speaking. For this reason, the larynx is often called the voice box. The vocal cords are composed of elastic fibers that help produce sound when air is forced between them. These sound waves are formed into words by the changing shapes of the pharynx and oral cavity and by using the tongue and lips.

Inferior to the larynx is the *trachea,* the passageway of air to the lungs. The trachea is a flexible cylindrical tube about one inch in diameter and approximately four inches in length. It is composed of 16 to 20 incomplete c–shaped rings of cartilage connected to one another by very elastic ligaments. The cartilage rings provide a semi–rigid support to the wall of the trachea, preventing it from collapsing inward. The trachea extends downward in front of the esophagus and into the thoracic cavity.

The *bronchial tree* consists of the branched airways extending from the trachea to the smallest respiratory unit in the lung. It begins with the left and right *primary bronchi* (pl.) Each primary bronchus enters a lung and then subdivides, forming left and right *secondary bronchi*. We see three secondary bronchi in the anatomical right lung. The secondary bronchi branch again and the *tertiary bronchi* become *bronchioles,* less than 1 mm in diameter. These bronchioles give off smaller *terminal bronchioles* that represent the end of the air-conducting pathway.

Each *respiratory bronchiole* supplies air to lobules. A lobule is a basic gas exchange complex composed of air cells, called *alveoli,* which are arranged in *alveolar sacs.* The walls of the air cells are surrounded by capillaries. *Capillaries* are networks of pulmonary *arterioles* and pulmonary *venules.* The walls of the capillaries are fused to the structurally similar walls of the alveoli. Oxygen and carbon dioxide rapidly diffuse through the walls of these microscopic cells. The blood readily absorbs the oxygen, and gives up the carbon dioxide which is quickly exhausted to the external atmosphere. These basic units make up most of the lung's volume. Nowhere in the body does the outside world, with all its creatures of microscopic dimension, have such an easy access to the protected interior cavities of the body as it does at the air/blood interfaces in the lungs.

lung (pneumon/o)	diaphragm
nasal cavity (nas/o)	pharynx (pharyng/o)
esophagus (esophag/o)	larynx (laryng/o)
breathe, breathing (pne/o)	air, gases (pneum/o)

trachea (trache/o)	pleura (pleur/o)

bronchus, (bronch/o), whether primary, secondary or tertiary parts of the bronchial tree.

41.
See above to help you identify the word root for each anatomical part. Then write a meaning for each of the following terms.

la rin jī′ tis
inflammation of the
   voice box

laryng/itis means _____

_____

plōōr ī′ tis
inflammation of the
   pleura

pleuritis means _____

_____;

fair ing′ gō plas tē
plastic surgery of the
   throat

pharyng/o/plasty means _____

_____.

42.
Look again at Illustration 10.3. Seeing the various parts will help you learn. What does laryng/o/cele mean? _____

la ring′ gō sēl
herniation of the voice
   box

_____.

laryngectomy
la rin jek′ tō mē

43.
Build a term meaning surgical removal of the voice box:

_____.

la ring′ gō skōp
instrument for
  examining the
  voice box

44.
Write a meaning for each of the following:

laryngoscope means _____

_____.

la ring′ gō spazm
spasm of the voice box

laryngospasm means _____

_____.

45.
See Illustration 10.3 again. _Trachea_ means windpipe. Write a brief definition for each of the following new terms:

trā kē ō rā′ jē ə
hemorrhage from the
  windpipe

tracheorrhagia _____

_____.

trā kē al′ jē ə
pain in the windpipe

trachealgia _____

_____.

trā kē os′ tō mē
a permanent opening
  into the windpipe

tracheostomy _____

_____.

46.
Write the word root and combining form for windpipe:

trache or trache/o

_____.

47.
A _bronchus_ is one of the major divisions of the windpipe. The bronchi (plural) direct the air into the lungs. Write a meaning for each of the following:

brong kos′ kō pē
looking into the
  bronchus

bronchoscopy _____

_____.

bron′ kō spazm
spasm of the bronchus

bronchospasm _____

_____.

brong kī′ tis
inflammation of the
  bronchus or bronchi

bronchitis _____

_____.

48.
The word root and combining form meaning major branches of the windpipe that open into the lungs is _____.

bronch, bronch/o

49.
Pleural means pertaining to the covering on the lungs. The pleural membrane completely covers the lungs and clings to it like plastic wrap. Only a few drops of thick fluid keep the lung and the pleura apart.

ploo rī′ tis
inflammation of the
    pleura

Pleuritis means _____

_____.

pleuralgia or
    pleurodynia
ploo ral′ jē ə
ploo rō din′ ē ə

50.
Pleurisy is another word for inflammation of the covering of the lungs. Build a term that means pain in the pleura:

_____.

ploo rō sen tē′ sis
puncture of the pleural
    space and removing
    the fluid

51.
Pleurisy may cause excessive fluid to collect within the space between the lung and the pleura. What do you think pleurocentesis means? _____

_____.

diaphragm
dī′ a fram

52.
Refer to Illustration 10.3 again. The musculomembranous wall separating the abdomen from the chest cavity is the _____.

in

53.
During inspiration the diaphragm contracts; it flattens out downward, permitting the lungs to move downward and fill with air. Inspiration is breathing _____.
                                        (in/out)

out

54.
During expiration the diaphragm relaxes. It resumes its inverted basin shape, squeezing the lungs and expelling the air out of the lungs. Expiration is breathing _____.
                                        (in/out)

diaphragm

55.
The organ largely responsible for inspiration and expiration is the _____.

hiccough, or hiccup
hik′ kof

56.
A sudden spasm of the diaphragm usually produces a giggle all around. It is called singultus. Can you guess what it means?
_____.

singultus sin gul′ tus	**57.** Another term for hiccough is _____.
hē mop′ ti sis spitting blood	**58.** *Ptysis* means spitting. What does hem/o/ptysis mean? _____ _____.
-ptysis	**59.** Hemoptysis means spitting blood (arising from hemorrhage of lar- ynx, trachea, bronchi, or lungs). Write the suffix meaning spitting, or spitting up. _____
hē ma tem′ a sis expelling blood from 　the stomach (vomiting blood)	What does hemat/emesis mean? _____ _____.
hem/o, hemat/o	**60.** Write the two combining forms for blood you just used in frames above. _____ and _____.
	61. Using either suffix, -ptysis or -emesis, build a medical term to express the following definitions:
hemoptysis	spitting blood from hemorrhage of the lungs is _____
hematemesis	expelling blood from the stomach is _____
rīn or ra′ jē a hemorrhage from the 　nose	**62.** *Epistaxis* means nosebleed. What does rhinorrhagia mean? _____.
epistaxis ep i stak′ sis rhinorrhagia	**63.** Two terms mean severe bleeding from the nose. They are _____ and _____.
spitting blood (arising 　from the larynx, 　trachea, bronchi, or 　lungs)	**64.** What does hemoptysis mean? _____ _____.
vomiting blood (from 　the stomach)	**65.** What does hematemesis mean? _____ _____.

epistaxis rhinorrhagia	66. Nasal hemorrhage is _____ or _____.

nyoo mat′ ik
pertaining to air or
   gases (or exchange
   of gases)
	67.
	Pneum/o, pneumat/o mean air, gases, or exchange of gases. What does pneumatic mean? _____
	_____.

brad ip nē′ a breathing very slowly	68. Pne/o relates to breathing. Do you remember what bradypnea means? _____
pne/o (nē ō)	69. The combining form referring to inhale and exhale, or in other words to breathe, is _____.

Pneum/o, pneumat/o are combining forms meaning air, gases, or exchange of gases. Explain what these terms mean:

an abnormal condition of air in a joint	Pneum/arthr/osis _____ _____
a condition of air in the heart	Pneumato/cardia _____ _____
air in the urine during or after urination	Pneumat/uria _____ _____
pneum–	What is the word root for air or gases? _____.
nyoo mol′ ō jē air or gases	70. Pneum/ology refers to the science of how the lungs exchange _____ or _____.
not breathing, breathing is absent	Apnea means _____.
pneumotherapy nyoo mō ther′ ə pē	71. Hydrotherapy means treatment with water. Build a term meaning treatment with (compressed) air: _____.
pneum/o pneumon/o	72. *Pneumon, pneumon/o* mean lung. At a quick glance you may confuse it with the root for air or gases. Write the combining forms for both: _____; _____. air or gases lung

73.

pneumonitis
nyōō mō nī′ tis

pneumonectomy
nyōō mōn ek′ tō mē

Pneumonia is a serious disease of the lung. Build a term for each of the following:
inflammation of the lung _____.
surgical removal of a lung _____.

74.

Drawing air into the lungs and pushing air out of the lungs is called breathing. The combining form referring to breathing is

pne/o (nē ō)   _____.

75.

nyōō mon′ ō graf

radiographic picture of the lungs (chest X ray)

Pneum/o/encephal/o/graphy means X ray examination of spaces within the brain. These X rays are taken following withdrawal of cerebrospinal fluid (via lumbar puncture) and replacement of it with injected air or gas. What is a pneumon/o/graph? _____
_____.

76.

breathing, breathe
air or gas
lung

Write a brief meaning for each of the following:
Pne/o _____.
Pneum/o or pneumat/o _____.
Pneumon/o _____.

77.

thorax
thor′ aks

Thorax encloses the chest cavity. It refers to the upper part of the trunk between the neck and the abdomen. The diaphragm separates the abdomen from the _____.

78.

thoracic cavity or
thorax

The organs of the digestive apparatus are enclosed in the abdomen. The chief organs of the circulatory and respiratory systems are located in the _____.

79.

thor a cot′ ə mē
incision into the chest cavity

thor a cō sen tē′ sis
puncture of the chest cavity to draw off fluid

Thorac and *thorac/o* are the word root and combining form referring to the chest cavity.

Thoracotomy means _____
_____.

Explain thoracocentesis: _____
_____.

hē mō thor′ aks
blood in the chest
   cavity

80.
Pneumothorax means air in the chest cavity. What does hemotho-
rax mean? _____.

81.
Let's conclude this unit with a review. Using the suggested answers,
complete each of the following brief definitions. Write your answer
in the space provided.

SUGGESTED ANSWERS:

bronchus(i)	pleura
diaphragm	trachea
larynx	singultus
pharynx	epistaxis

larynx
bronchi
epistaxis
trachea
singultus
pharynx
pleura
diaphragm

voice box, _____.
main branches of the windpipe, _____.
severe nosebleed, _____.
windpipe, _____.
hiccough, _____.
throat, _____.
tough film enveloping the lungs, _____.
muscle controlling breathing, _____.

82.
Try that again.

SUGGESTED ANSWERS:

apneic	hemoptysis
pneumothorax	rhinoplasty
pneumonogram	pneumonia
nasal	pleurodynia

pneumonia
hemoptysis
pneumonogram
pneumothorax
nasal
rhinoplasty
pleurodynia
apneic

serious lung condition, _____.
spitting blood (arising from trachea), _____.
X ray of the lung(s), _____.
collection of air in the chest cavity, _____.
pertaining to the nose, _____.
a "nose job," _____.
pain in the pleura, _____.
pertaining to absence of breathing, _____.

83.

Here's one last exercise to show how far you have come! For each area of medical concern, write the term describing a practicing specialist

	AREA OF MEDICAL CONCERN	SPECIALIST
Pathologist	Bodily changes in structure and function due to disease	_____
Psychiatrist	Mental illness	_____
Dermatologist	Skin and its diseases	_____
Gynecologist	Diseases of women	_____
Cardiologist	Diseases of the heart	_____
Neurologist	Nervous system diseases	_____
Pediatrician	Childhood illnesses	_____
Obstetrician	Pregnancy and childbirth	_____
Ophthalmologist	Diseases of the eye	_____
Urologist	Conditions of urogenitals	_____

84.

Try it again. Describe the area of medical concern for these specialists.

	SPECIALIST	AREA OF MEDICAL CONCERN
Bones and muscles	Orthopedist	_____
Pregnancy and childbirth	Obstetrician	_____
Old age, aging	Geriatrician	_____
Causes of epidemics	Epidemiologist	_____
Skilled diagnosing	Diagnostician	_____
Anesthesia and pain	Anesthesiologist	_____
Urinary and genitals	Urologist	_____
Tumors and treatment	Oncologist	_____
Ear, nose, throat, and voice box	Otorhinopharyngo-laryngologist	_____

85.

Here are 50 more medical terms you have worked with in Unit 10. Don't forget to pronounce each one carefully before taking the final Unit 10 Self-Test.

apnea (ap′ nē ə)

bradypnea (brad ip nē′ ə)

blepharedema (blef′ ar ə dē′ mä)

blepharorrhaphy (blef ar ōr′ ā fē)

blepharoptosis (blef ar op tō′ sis)

bronchitis (brong kī′ tis)
bronchoscopy (brong kos′ kō pē)
corectasia (kōr ek tā′ zē ə)
corectopia (kōr ek tō′ pē ə)
coreometer (kōr ē om′ e ter)
coreoplasty (kōr′ ē ō plas tē)
corneal (kor′ nē al)
cyclokerititis (sī′ klō ker i tī′ tis)
cycloplegia (sī klō plē′ jē ə)
diaphragm (dī′ a fram)
diplopia (di plō′ pē ə)
epistaxis (ep i stak′ sis)
hemoptysis (hē mop′ ti sis)
iridectomy (ir i dek′ tō mē)
iridocele (ir id ō sēl)
iridoplegia (ir id ō plē′ jē ə)
iritis (ī rī′ tis)
keratome (ker′ ə tōm)
keratoplasty (ker′ ə tō plas tē)
keratoscleritis
    (ker′ ə tō skler ī′ tis)
keratotomy (ker a tōt′ ō mē)
laryngeal (la rin′ jē al)
laryngospasm
    (la ring′ gō spazm)
nasolacrimal (nā zō lak′ ri məl)
nasopharyngitis
    (nā′ zō fair in jī′ tis)

ophthalmalgia
    (of′ thal mal′ jē a)
ophthalmoscope
    (of thal′ mō skōp)
pharyngitis (fair in jī′ tis)
pharyngotomy
    (fair in got′ ō mē)
pleuralgia (ploo ral′ jē ə)
pleurisy (ploor′ i sē)
pleurocentesis
    (ploor′ ō sen tē′ sis)
pneumohemothorax
    (nyoo mō hē mō thōr′ aks)
pneumonia (nyoo mō′ nē ə)
retinitis (ret i nī′ tis)
retinopathy (ret i nop′ ə thē)
retinoscopy (ret i nos′ kō pē)
rhinoplasty (ri′ nō plas tē)
sclerectomy (skler ek′ tō mē)
sclerotome (skler′ ə tōm)
singultus (sing gul′ tus)
tracheorrhagia
    (trā kē ō rāj′ jē ə)
tracheostomy
    (trā kē os′ tō mē)
thorax (thor′ aks)
thoracocentesis
    (thôr′ ə kō sen tē′ sis)

Unit 10 Self-Test

Part 1

From the list on the right, select the correct meaning for each of the following often used medical terms.

_____ 1. Pneumonectomy

_____ 2. Keratoscleritis

_____ 3. Pleurocentesis

_____ 4. Corectasia

_____ 5. Pleuralgia

_____ 6. Blepharedema

_____ 7. Hemoptysis

_____ 8. Ophthalmologist

_____ 9. Nasomental

_____ 10. Iridoplegia

_____ 11. Tracheorrhagia

_____ 12. Keratome

_____ 13. Epistaxis

_____ 14. Retinoid

_____ 15. Bronchitis

a. Nosebleed

b. Spitting blood

c. Pertaining to nose and chin

d. Stretching (dilation) of the pupil

e. Puncture of the pleural space to remove fluid

f. Pain of the pleura

g. Instrument to cut the cornea

h. Paralysis of the iris

i. Inflammation of cornea and sclera

j. Resembling the retina

k. Swollen eyelids due to fluid in the tissues

l. Physician who specializes in the study of eye diseases

m. Hemorrhage from the trachea

n. Inflammation of the bronchi

o. Surgical removal of a lung

Part 2

Write the medical term for each of the following brief definitions.

1. Air in the chest cavity _____
2. Pertaining to nose and tears _____
3. Incision into the throat _____
4. Hiccough _____
5. Instrument to examine the eye _____
6. Plastic surgery of the cornea _____
7. Double vision _____
8. Drooping eyelid _____
9. Pain in the covering of the lung _____
10. Permanent opening into the windpipe _____
11. Inflammation of the iris _____
12. Spasm of the voice box _____
13. Pertaining to the cornea _____
14. Nosebleed _____
15. Very fast breathing _____

ANSWERS

Part 1	Part 2
1. o	1. Pneumothorax
2. i	2. Nasolacrimal
3. e	3. Pharyngotomy
4. d	4. Singultus
5. f	5. Ophthalmoscope
6. k	6. Keratoplasty
7. b	7. Diplopia
8. l	8. Blepharoptosis
9. c	9. Pleurodynia
10. h	10. Tracheostomy
11. m	11. Iritis
12. g	12. Laryngospasm
13. a	13. Corneal
14. j	14. Epistaxis
15. n	15. Tachypnea

Review Sheets

Unit 1: Review Sheet

Part 1

Cover the column of words on the right. In the space provided write the meaning of each word part listed in the left column. Check your answers.

Word Part	Meaning	(Hide This Column)
acr/o–	_____	extremity
megal/o–	_____	enlargement
dermat/o–	_____	skin
cyan/o–	_____	blue
derm/o–	_____	skin
leuk/o–	_____	white
–itis	_____	inflammation
cardi/o–	_____	heart
gastr/o–	_____	stomach
cyt/o–	_____	cell
–ologist	_____	one who studies
–algia	_____	pain
–ectomy	_____	excision
–otomy	_____	incision
–ostomy	_____	new opening
duoden/o–	_____	duodenum
electr/o–	_____	electricity
–ology	_____	study of
–osis	_____	condition of
–tome	_____	instrument that cuts
gram/o–	_____	record
eti/o–	_____	cause of
path/o–	_____	disease

Now, do Part 2.

Part 2

Cover the word parts in the right-hand column. In the space provided write a suffix or word part that expresses the meaning of each word in the left column. Check your answers.

Meaning	Word Part	(Hide This Column)
record	_____	gram/o-
one who studies (suffix)	_____	-ologist
enlargement	_____	megal/o-
electric	_____	electr/o-
white	_____	leuk/o-
incision into (suffix)	_____	-otomy
blue	_____	cyan/o-
instrument that cuts (suffix)	_____	-tome
stomach	_____	gastr/o-
extremity	_____	acr/o-
(abnormal) condition of (suffix)	_____	-osis
changes due to disease	_____	path/o-
new opening formed (suffix)	_____	-ostomy
skin	_____	dermat/o-, dermat
study of (suffix)	_____	-ology
heart	_____	cardi/o-
excision (suffix)	_____	-ectomy
inflammation of (suffix)	_____	-itis
duodenum	_____	duoden/o-
pain (suffix)	_____	-algia
cell	_____	cyt/o-
cause of	_____	eti/o-

Unit 2: Review Sheet

Part 1

Cover the column of words on the right. In the space provided write the meaning of the word parts listed in the left column. Check your answers.

Word Part	Meaning	(Hide This Column)
aden/o-	_____	gland
carcin/o-	_____	cancer
malac/o-	_____	soft, softened
-oid	_____	resembling
laryng/o-	_____	larynx
cephal/o-	_____	head
hyper-	_____	excessive, more than normal
-cele	_____	herniation
ost/o-, oste/o-	_____	bone
arthr/o-	_____	joint
chondr/o-	_____	cartilage
cost/o-	_____	rib
lip/o-	_____	fat
inter-	_____	between
dent/o-, dont/o	_____	tooth
-emesis	_____	vomiting
-oma	_____	tumor
-plast/o, -plast/y	_____	repair
hypo-	_____	under, less than normal
troph/o-	_____	development
morph/o-	_____	structure and form
muc/o-	_____	mucus
onc/o-	_____	tumor
hist/o-	_____	tissue(s)
en-, endo-	_____	inside, within
ex-, exo-	_____	out, completely outside

Part 2

Cover the column on the right while you work. In the space provided, write the word part or combining form that matches the definition listed in the left column.

Meaning	Word Part	(Hide This Column)
rib	_____	cost/o–
larynx	_____	laryng/o–
development	_____	troph/o–
cancer	_____	carcin/o–
repair (suffix)	_____	–plast/o(/y)
tooth	_____	dent/o–, dont/o
mucus	_____	muc/o–
under, less than normal	_____	hypo–
herniation (suffix)	_____	–cele
soft, softened	_____	malac/o–
gland	_____	aden/o–
tumor (suffix)	_____	–oma
bone	_____	oste/o–
vomiting (suffix)	_____	–emesis
head	_____	cephal/o–
joint	_____	arthr/o–
between (prefix)	_____	inter–
resembling (suffix)	_____	–oid
fat	_____	lip/o–
inside, within (prefix)	_____	en–, endo–
cartilage	_____	chondr/o–
excessive, more than normal (prefix)	_____	hyper–
tissue	_____	hist/o–
structure and form	_____	morph/o–
tumor(s)	_____	onc/o–
out, completely outside (prefix)	_____	ex–, exo–

Unit 3: Review Sheet

Part 1

Cover the column of words on the right. In the space provided write the meaning of each word part listed in the left column. Check your answers.

Word Part	Meaning	(Hide This Column)
cyst/o–	_____	bladder
–ar	_____	pertaining to
crani/o–	_____	cranium (skull)
dipl/o–	_____	double
ab–	_____	away from
cocc/i–	_____	coccus
metr/o, meter–	_____	measure
py/o–	_____	pus
–genesis, gen/o–	_____	produce, originate
–orrhea	_____	flow
ot/o–	_____	ear
–centesis	_____	puncture
rhin/o–	_____	nose
lith/o–	_____	stone or calculus
hydro–	_____	water
chol/e–	_____	gall, bile
thorac/o–	_____	thorax or chest
pelv/i–	_____	pelvis
ad–	_____	toward
abdomin/o–	_____	abdomen
therap/o–	_____	treatment
cephal/o–	_____	head, cranium
phob/ia	_____	fear
cardi/o	_____	heart

Now, do Part 2.

Part 2

Cover the word parts on the right. In the space provided write a term that expresses the meaning of each word in the left column. Check your answers.

Meaning	Word Part	(Hide This Column)
water, watery fluid	_____	hydro-
flow, discharge (suffix)	_____	-orrhea
abnormal fear	_____	phob/ia
double, pairs	_____	dipl/o-
head	_____	cephal/o
pelvis	_____	pelv/i-
gall, bile	_____	chol/e-
nose	_____	rhin/o-
puncture of a cavity (suffix)	_____	-centesis
pus	_____	py/o-
treatment	_____	therap/o-
toward the midline (prefix)	_____	ad-
produce, originate (suffix, prefix)	_____	-genesis, gen/o-
bladder	_____	cyst/o-
coccus	_____	cocc/i-, cocc/o
measure	_____	metr/o-, meter-
stone or calculus	_____	lith/o-
ear	_____	ot/o-
thorax or chest	_____	thorac/o-
cranium (skull)	_____	crani/o-
away from the midline (prefix)	_____	ab-
abdomen	_____	abdomin/o-

Unit 4: Review Sheet

Part 1

Cover the right-hand column. Write the meaning of each word or word part in the left column. Be sure to check your answers.

Word/Word Part	Meaning	(Hide This Column)
-peps/ia	_____	digestion
neur/o-	_____	nerve
blast/o-	_____	immature cell form, germ cell
a-, an-	_____	without
angi/o-	_____	vessel
-spasm	_____	twitching, spasm
scler/o-	_____	hard, hardened
-tachy	_____	fast
aneurysm	_____	ballooning-out vessel
fibr/o-	_____	fibrous, fiber
lys/o-	_____	destruction, dissolution
pne/o-	_____	breathe, breathing
arteri/o-	_____	artery
men/o-	_____	menses, menstruation
hemat/o-, hemo-	_____	blood
kinesi/o-	_____	movement
spermat/o-	_____	spermatozoon, spermatozoa (plural)
oophor/o-	_____	ovary
-pexy	_____	fixation
salping/o-	_____	fallopian tube
dys-	_____	bad, painful, difficult
hyster/o-	_____	uterus
-ptosis	_____	prolapse, drooping
-brady	_____	slow
anomaly	_____	irregularity, breaks the rule
ur/o-	_____	urine

(Continued on next page)

nephr/o–	_____	kidney
pyel/o–	_____	renal pelvis
ureter/o–	_____	ureter
–orrhaphy	_____	to suture, repair
urethr/o–	_____	urethra
–orrhagia	_____	hemorrhage
colp/o–	_____	vagina
crypt/o–	_____	hidden
orchid/o–	_____	testis, testes (plural)
hernia	_____	protrusion through cavity wall

Part 2

Meaning	Word/Word Part	(Hide This Column)
artery	_____	arteri/o-
vessel	_____	angi/o-
uterus	_____	hyster/o-
movement	_____	kinesi/o-
destruction, dissolution	_____	lys/o-
blood	_____	hemat/o-, hem/o-
protrusion through cavity wall	_____	hernia
urine	_____	ur/o-
hard, hardening	_____	scler/o-
slow (prefix)	_____	brady-
fallopian tube	_____	salping/o-
muscle	_____	my/o-
without (prefix)	_____	a-, an-
nerve	_____	neur/o-
surgical fixation (suffix)	_____	-pexy
germ cell (immature)	_____	blast/o-
ballooning-out vessel	_____	aneurysm
ovary	_____	oophor/o-
breathe	_____	pne/o-
digestion	_____	-peps/ia
prolapse, drooping	_____	-ptosis
bad, painful, difficult (prefix)	_____	dys-
spermatozoa (pl.)	_____	spermat/o-
fibrous, fiber	_____	fibr/o-
twitching (suffix)	_____	-spasm
fast, rapid (prefix)	_____	tachy-
hemorrhage (suffix)	_____	-orrhagia
renal pelvis	_____	pyel/o-
vagina	_____	colp/o-
ureter	_____	ureter/o-
kidney	_____	nephr/o-
irregularity, breaks the rule	_____	anomaly

(Continued on next page)

urethra	_____	urethr/o-
to suture, repair (suffix)	_____	-orrhaphy
hidden	_____	crypt/o-
testes (pl.)	_____	orchid/o-
menses, menstruation	_____	men/o-

Congratulations!

Unit 5: Review Sheet

Part 1

Cover the right-hand column. Write the meaning of each word or word part in the left column. Be sure to check your answers.

Word/ Word Part	Meaning	(Hide This Column)
stomat/o–	_____	mouth
gloss/o–	_____	tongue
cheil/o–	_____	lips
gingiv/o–	_____	gums
esophag/o–	_____	esophagus
enter/o–	_____	small intestine
–scope	_____	instrument to look, examine
col/o–	_____	colon
rect/o–	_____	rectum
proct/o–	_____	anus and rectum
hepat/o–	_____	liver
pancreat/o–	_____	pancreas
clys/o, –clysis	_____	wash, irrigate
–ectasia	_____	dilation, stretching
–spasm	_____	twitching, cramping
dent/o–	_____	teeth, tooth
toxin	_____	poison, poisoning
hypo–	_____	under, beneath
hyper–	_____	excessive
–algia	_____	pain, ache
–osis	_____	abnormal, diseased condition
–ostomy	_____	surgery to form a new opening (permanent)
–otomy	_____	incision into
–ectomy	_____	surgical removal of
–pexy	_____	surgical fixation of a part in its normal place

Part 2

Meaning	Word/Word Part	(Hide This Column)
cramping, twitching		spasm
liver		hepat/o–
excessive (prefix)		hyper–
small intestine		enter/o–
surgical incision into (suffix)		–otomy
surgery to form a new opening (suffix)		–ostomy
pertaining to teeth		dental
rectum and anus		proct/o–
lips		cheil/o–
wash, irrigate (suffix)		–clysis
esophagus		esophag/o–
colon		col/o–
gums		gingiv/o–
mouth		stomat/o–
pain, ache (suffix)		–algia
dilation, stretching (a suffix)		–ectasia
pancreas		pancreat/o–
rectum		rect/o–
tongue		gloss/o–
surgical fixation of a part in normal place (suffix)		–pexy
look, examine (suffix)		–scopy

Unit 6: Review Sheet

Part 1

Cover the right-hand column. Write the meaning of each word or word part listed in the left-hand column in the space provided. Be sure to check your answers.

Word/ Word Part	Meaning	(Hide This Column)
phleb/o-	_____	vein
dys-	_____	bad, difficult, painful
-orrhexis	_____	rupture, bursting apart
-esthesia	_____	sensation, feeling
fibrillation	_____	very rapid heartbeat
-algesia	_____	sensation of pain
phas/o-	_____	speech
thrombosis	_____	occlusion of a blood vessel by a blood clot
-tripsy	_____	surgical crushing
plas/o-	_____	formation, development
syn-, sym,	_____	together as one
a-, an-	_____	without, absent
embolus	_____	foreign particle floating in bloodstream
dactyl/o-	_____	fingers, toes, digits
cardiac arrest	_____	cessation of heartbeat
-emia	_____	blood
embolism	_____	vessel occluded, blocked by an embolus
myel/o-	_____	spinal cord, or bone marrow
poly-	_____	many
micro-	_____	very small, microscopic
defibrillation	_____	restoration of regular heartbeat (often with electric shock)
thrombus	_____	blood clot in the bloodstream

Part 2

Meaning	Word/Word Part	(Hide This Column)
a blood clot in the bloodstream	_____	thrombus
sensation, feeling	_____	–esthesia
speech	_____	phas/o–
sensation of pain	_____	–algesia
vein	_____	phleb/o–
vessel occluded by an embolus	_____	embolism
restoration of regular heartbeat often by electric shock	_____	defibrillation
foreign particle circulating in the bloodstream	_____	embolus
formation, development in the sense of shaping, molding	_____	plas/o–
rupture, bursting apart (suffix)	_____	–orrhexis
bad, difficult, painful (prefix)	_____	dys–
surgical crushing (suffix)	_____	–tripsy
very, very small (prefix)	_____	micro–
large, seen by human eye (prefix)	_____	macro–
bone marrow or spinal cord	_____	myel/o–
finger or toe, digit	_____	dactyl/o–
many (prefix)	_____	poly–
together as one (prefix)	_____	syn–, sym–
very fast heartbeat	_____	fibrillation
blood (suffix)	_____	–emia

Unit 7: Review Sheet

Part 1

Word/ Word Part	Meaning	(Hide This Column)
edema	_____	fluid in the tissues
chronic	_____	long, drawn-out disease
syndrome	_____	symptoms occur together
prognosis	_____	prediction of course and outcome of disease
acute	_____	pertaining to severe symptom, rapid onset, short course
paroxysmal	_____	pertaining to sudden periodic attack
diagnosis	_____	identification of disease
tinnitus	_____	ringing in the ear
malaise	_____	vague sensation of not feeling well
vertigo	_____	sensation of turning around in space
anorexia	_____	loss of appetite
symptom	_____	perceived change in body or functions
pyrexia	_____	feverishness
mortality	_____	pertaining to being mortal
morbidity	_____	pertaining to being diseased
hypertrophy	_____	overdevelopment
atrophy	_____	wasting away, shrinking of an organ
systemic	_____	pertaining to the whole body, all systems

(Continued on next page)

vital signs	_____	T, P, and R
peripheral	_____	pertaining to the outside surface of the body
chlor/o–	_____	green
melan/o–	_____	black
erythr/o–	_____	red
xanth/o–	_____	yellow
prophylactic	_____	pertaining to prevention of disease
prodromal	_____	pertaining to phase of disease before symptoms
nausea	_____	seasickness, inclined to vomit
palliative	_____	pertaining to relief of symptoms, not cure
against (prefix)	_____	anti–
dyspnea	_____	difficult, painful breathing
hypothermia	_____	subnormal temperature, below 90°F

Part 2

Meaning	Word/Word Part	(Hide This Column)
symptoms occur together	_____	syndrome
prediction of course and outcome of disease	_____	prognosis
pertaining to severe symptom, rapid onset, short course	_____	acute
wasting away, shrinking of an organ	_____	atrophy
pertaining to the whole body, all systems	_____	systemic
T, P, and R	_____	vital signs
fluid in the tissues	_____	edema
long, drawn-out disease	_____	chronic
pertaining to sudden periodic attack	_____	paroxysmal
identification of disease	_____	diagnosis
ringing in the ear	_____	tinnitus
vague sensation of not feeling well	_____	malaise
sensation of turning around in space	_____	vertigo
loss of appetite	_____	anorexia
perceived change in body or functions	_____	symptom
statistic pertaining to being diseased	_____	morbidity
pertaining to relief of symptoms, not cure	_____	palliative
fever	_____	pyret/o-, pyrexia

(Continued on next page)

pertaining to phase of disease before symptoms	_____	prodromal
pertaining to prevention of disease	_____	prophylactic
yellow	_____	xanth/o-
red	_____	erythr/o-
seasickness, inclined to vomit	_____	nausea
black	_____	melan/o-
green	_____	chlor/o-
pertaining to the outside surface of the body	_____	peripheral
breathing reaches a climax, then ceases before starting again	_____	Cheyne-Stokes respiration
difficult, painful breathing	_____	dyspnea
overdevelopment	_____	hypertrophy
statistic pertaining to being mortal	_____	mortality
feverishness	_____	pyret/o-, pyrexia
loss of appetite	_____	anorexia
symptoms occurring before the onset of the disease	_____	prodrome

Unit 8: Review Sheet

Part 1

Word/ Word Part	Meaning	(Hide This Column)
supra–, super–	_____	above, over
cyst	_____	closed sac containing fluid
neoplasm	_____	new tissue growth, no purpose
lesion	_____	unhealthy, diseased tissue
infra–	_____	below, beneath, under
ectopic	_____	outside the normal place
ect/o–	_____	outside
papule, papula	_____	raised red spot, pimple
peri–, circum–	_____	around, about, nearby
ventral	_____	on or near the belly
epi–	_____	over, upon, surrounding
distal	_____	point farthest from trunk
dorsal	_____	on or near the back
epigastric	_____	area of the belly over the stomach
proximal	_____	point nearest to the trunk
papilloma	_____	nipple-shaped tumor on skin
lateral	_____	farther from the midline
infiltration	_____	slipping into and between normal cells
sub–, hypo–	_____	below, beneath
excrescence	_____	outgrowth, wart
medial	_____	nearer to the midline

(Continued on next page)

papilla	_____	small, nipple–like protuberance
condyloma	_____	perianal wartlike growth
benign	_____	not spreading, not malignant
end/o–	_____	inner, inside
malignant	_____	bad kind, threatening death
tumor, neoplasm	_____	new, abnormal tissue growth
metastasis	_____	cells spread to new location
polyp	_____	tumor on a little foot, or stem
circumscribed	_____	as a line drawn around, edge
mes/o–	_____	middle

Part 2

Meaning	Word/Word Part	(Hide This Column)
new, abnormal tissue growth	_____	tumor
cells spread to new location	_____	metastasis
middle (prefix)	_____	mes/o–
point nearest to the trunk	_____	proximal
perianal wartlike growth	_____	condyloma
not spreading, not malignant	_____	benign
inner, inside (prefix)	_____	end/o–
bad kind, threatening death	_____	malignant
closed sac containing fluid	_____	cyst
as a line drawn around, edge	_____	circumscribed
area of the belly over the stomach	_____	epigastric
new tissue growth, no purpose	_____	neoplasm
unhealthy, diseased tissue	_____	lesion
beneath the patella	_____	subpatellar, infrapatellar
outside the normal place	_____	ectopic
raised red spot, pimple	_____	papule, papula
around, circular (prefix)	_____	circum–
on or near the belly	_____	ventral
above the pubic arch	_____	suprapubic
below, beneath, under (prefix)	_____	infra–, sub–, hypo–
on or near the back	_____	dorsal

(Continued on next page)

slipping into and between normal cells   —————————————   infiltration

tumor on a little foot   —————————————   polyp

over, surrounding (prefix)   —————————————   epi-

around, about, nearby (prefix)   —————————————   peri-

under the skin   —————————————   hypodermic

point farthest from trunk   —————————————   distal

nipple-shaped tumor on skin   —————————————   papilloma

farther from the midline   —————————————   lateral

removal and examination of living tissue   —————————————   biopsy

Unit 9: Review Sheet

Part 1

Word/ Word Part	Meaning	(Hide This Column)
conception	_____	union of ovum and spermatozoon
ovum	_____	female egg cell
peritoneum	_____	thin membrane that coats the viscera and lines the abdominal wall
secundi-	_____	second
fetus	_____	developing child in utero
spermatozoon	_____	male germ cell
parturition	_____	labor and delivery of term pregnancy
multi-	_____	many
nulli-	_____	none
postpartum	_____	time period after giving birth
mastopathy	_____	breast disease
hysterorrhexis	_____	rupture of uterus (life threatening)
metratrophy	_____	uterine atrophy
antepartum	_____	time period before labor
prenatal	_____	before childbirth
oligo- hydramnios	_____	scanty amount of amniotic fluid
mamm/o-, mast/o-	_____	breast
amniot/o-	_____	amnion (sac for fetus and fluid)
-atrophy	_____	wasting of an organ or part
primipara	_____	a woman who has given birth for the first time

(Continued on next page)

–dynia	_____	pain, painful
–mania	_____	madness
–phobia	_____	excessive fear
–gravida	_____	heavy with child; a pregnant woman
men/o–	_____	menses, menstruation
involution	_____	process of uterus returning to nonpregnant state
climacteric	_____	change of life period
placenta	_____	organ that nourishes fetus in utero
gynecomastia	_____	enlarged breasts in a male
puerperium	_____	period after childbirth; involution takes place
pudenda	_____	female external genitals
gestation	_____	another term for pregnancy
amniocentesis	_____	puncture of amniotic sac and removal of fluid
perineum	_____	pelvic floor; region from vaginal lip to anus in female

Part 2

Meaning	Word/Word Part	(Hide This Column)
female external genitals	_____	pudenda
menses, menstruation	_____	men/o-
madness (suffix)	_____	-mania
female egg cell	_____	ovum
wasting of an organ or part (suffix)	_____	-atrophy
another term for pregnancy	_____	gestation
puncture of amniotic sac and removal of fluid	_____	amniocentesis
enlarged breasts in a male	_____	gynecomastia
breast disease	_____	mastopathy
breast (2 combining forms)	_____	mast/o-, mamm/o-
none (prefix)	_____	nulli-
many (prefix)	_____	multi-
developing child in utero	_____	fetus
male germ cell	_____	spermatozoon
cessation of menses	_____	menopause
pregnant woman, first time	_____	primigravida
incision of vagina and pelvic outlet	_____	episiotomy
excessive fear (prefix)	_____	phobia-
pain, painful (suffix)	_____	-dynia, -algia
process of uterus returning to nonpregnant state	_____	involution
rupture of uterus (life threatening)	_____	hysterorrhexis
woman who has given birth to a living child	_____	para
pelvic floor; region from vaginal lip to anus in female	_____	perineum

(Continued on next page)

period after childbirth; involution takes place	_____	puerperium
amnion (sac for fetus and fluid)	_____	amni/o-, amniot/o-
organ that nourishes fetus in utero	_____	placenta
few, little, scanty (prefix)	_____	oligo-
before labor	_____	antepartum
change of life period	_____	climacteric
physician specialist in diseases of women	_____	gynecologist
before (prefix)	_____	pre-
after (prefix)	_____	post-
new, recent (prefix)	_____	neo-
labor and delivery of term pregnancy	_____	parturition
X ray examination of breast	_____	mammography
thin membrane that coats viscera and abdominal wall	_____	peritoneum
union of ovum and spermatozoon	_____	conception
uterine atrophy	_____	metratrophy
pain, painful (suffix)	_____	-dynia, -algia
heavy with child; a pregnant woman	_____	gravida

Unit 10: Review Sheet

Part 1

Word/ Word Part	Meaning	(Hide This Column)
nas/o–	_____	nose
blephar/o–	_____	eyelid
scler/o–	_____	hard white coat of the eye
pharyng/o–	_____	pharynx, throat
ir, irid/o–	_____	iris, donut-shaped color of the eye
dipl/o–	_____	double, paired
laryng/o–	_____	larynx, voice box
pneumon/o–	_____	lung
bronch/o–	_____	bronchus(i), branches of the trachea
ophthalm/o–	_____	eye
retin/o–	_____	retina, complex membrane on the inside back surface of the eyeball
pleur/o–	_____	pleura, covering on the lungs
core–, core/o–	_____	pupil, circular opening in the center of the eye
pne/o–	_____	breathing, breathe
lacrim/o–	_____	tear, tears
ment/o–	_____	chin
kerat/o–, corne/o–	_____	cornea, transparent covering of anterior one-sixth of the eye
–opia	_____	suffix meaning vision
thorac/o–	_____	thorax, chest
cycl/o–	_____	ciliary body, controls the shape of the iris
pneum/o–	_____	air, gases
trache/o–	_____	windpipe, trachea
singultus	_____	hiccup, hiccough

(Continued on next page)

hemoptysis   _____   spitting of blood
                                                   derived from the
                                                   lungs, bronchi

diaphragm   _____   musculo–membranous
                                                   wall separating the
                                                   abdomen from the
                                                   thorax

epistaxis   _____   nosebleed

Part 2

Meaning	Word/Word Part	(Hide This Column)
nose	_____	nas/o–
breathing, breathe	_____	pne/o–
iris	_____	ir–, irid/o–
larynx, voice box	_____	laryng/o–
cornea, transparent anterior covering of one-sixth of the eye	_____	kerat/o–, corne/o–
nosebleed	_____	epistaxis
spitting blood derived from the lungs, trachea	_____	hemoptysis
suffix meaning vision	_____	–opia
musculomembranous wall separating the abdomen from the thorax	_____	diaphragm
air, gases	_____	pneum/o–
retina, complex membrane on the inside back surface of the eyeball	_____	retin/o–
pleura, covering on the lungs	_____	pleur/o–
eyelid	_____	blephar/o–
tear, tears	_____	lacrim/o–
windpipe, trachea	_____	trache/o–
pupil, circular opening in the center of the eye	_____	cor–, core–, core/o–
hard white coat of the eye	_____	scler/o–
pharynx, throat	_____	pharyng/o–
bronchus(i), branches of the trachea	_____	bronch/o–
lung	_____	pneumon/o–
ciliary body, controls shape of the iris	_____	cycl/o–

(Continued on next page)

thorax, chest	_____	thorac/o–
chin	_____	ment/o–
double, paired	_____	dipl/o–
eye	_____	ophthalm/o–
hiccup, hiccough	_____	singultus

Congratulations on finishing your lessons.
Take the other Final Test after some rest and relaxation.

Final Self-Test I

Instructions

The following two tests will show you how much you have learned about medical terminology. Many of the words on the tests will be new to you; however, using the word parts and the word-building system you have learned, you should be able to give the meaning for all of them. Try these tests and see how well you do. You may want to take one test before reading the book and the other after you finish the book. The comparison will show even more clearly how much medical terminology you have learned.

Each test consists of 50 medical terms. For each term, write out a definition in your own words. Then compare your answers with those following the test. Your definition should include all of the ideas (though not necessarily in the exact words) as the definitions on the answer page.

1. Tachypnea _____
2. Oophoritis _____
3. Pyelonephrosis _____
4. Pathogenic _____
5. Bradycardia _____
6. Cycloparalysis _____
7. Glossoplegia _____
8. Megalodontia _____
9. Ophthalmoscopy _____
10. Bronchopneumonogram _____
11. Mammopexy _____
12. Cystocele _____
13. Cephalometer _____
14. Herniorrhaphy _____

15. Hyperthyroidism _____

16. Bronchiectasis _____

17. Mastodynia _____

18. Xanthemia _____

19. Symptomatology _____

20. Etiology _____

21. Kinesialgia _____

22. Fibroosteoma _____

23. Anuria _____

24. Lipochondroma _____

25. Costectomy _____

26. Ureteroenterostomy _____

27. Metrorrhagia _____

28. Paranephritis _____

29. Blepharoptosis _____

30. Erythrocyte _____

31. Perianal _____

32. Endocarditis _____

33. Lymphadenoid _____

34. Thoracolumbar _____

35. Corneoiritis _____

36. Hysterorrhexis _____

37. Thrombogenesis _____

38. Hematemesis _____

39. Lithotripsy _____

40. Oligohydramnios _____

41. Prostatic hypertrophy _____

42. Hemoptysis _____

43. Dorsalgia _____

44. Endocranial _____

45. Parturition _____

46. Adenocarcinoma _____

47. Esophagogastrostomy _____

48. Enterohepatitis _____

49. Malaise _____

50. Dyspnea _____

Answers to Final Self-Test I

1. rapid breathing
2. inflammation of an ovary
3. condition (abnormal or diseased) of the pelvis of the kidney
4. that which is capable of causing disease
5. slow heart rate
6. paralysis of the ciliary body
7. paralysis of the tongue
8. excessively large teeth
9. examination of the interior of the eye
10. X ray of the bronchi and lungs
11. surgical fixation of a breast to its normal position
12. hernia of the bladder
13. instrument for measuring the head
14. suturing (repair) of a hernia
15. condition caused by excessive secretion of the thyroid glands
16. dilatation of the bronchi
17. painful breast
18. yellow pigment (color) in the blood
19. the study (science) of disease symptoms
20. the study of causes of disease
21. painful muscular movement
22. tumor of bone and fibrous connective tissue
23. absence of urine
24. tumor of cartilaginous and fatty tissue
25. excision of a rib or ribs
26. make a permanent opening between the ureter and intestine
27. uterine hemorrhage
28. inflammation of tissues around (surrounding) the kidney
29. drooping of an eyelid
30. red blood cell
31. of or pertaining to around the anus
32. inflammation of the inside (lining) of the heart
33. resembling a lymph gland
34. of or pertaining to the chest (thorax) and lower back (lumbar)
35. inflammation of the iris and cornea
36. rupture of the uterus
37. formation (development) of a clot (thrombus)
38. vomiting blood
39. crushing removal of a stone
40. scanty amniotic fluid
41. pertaining to enlargement of the prostate
42. spitting blood (from trachea, bronchi, or lungs)
43. pain in the back
44. of, or pertaining to, the inside of the head
45. labor and childbirth
46. malignant tumor of a gland
47. making a new opening (permanent) between the esophagus and the stomach
48. inflammation of the liver and intestine
49. vague sensation of not feeling well
50. difficult or painful breathing

Final Self-Test II

1. Mastoptosis _____
2. Epistaxis _____
3. Amenorrhea _____
4. Antipyretic _____
5. Nephrolith _____
6. Enterectasia _____
7. Paroxysmal _____
8. Encephalorrhagia _____
9. Craniocele _____
10. Anorexia _____
11. Gingivoglossitis _____
12. Cholecystitis _____
13. Abdominalgia _____
14. Arteriospasm _____
15. Adenosclerosis _____
16. Duodenohepatic _____
17. Endobronchoscopy _____
18. Iridoplegia _____
19. Tracheostomy _____
20. Syndactyly _____
21. Phleborrhexis _____
22. Cryptorchidism _____
23. Thromboid _____

24. Electroencephalogram _____

25. Myelodysplasia _____

26. Singultus _____

27. Intercostal _____

28. Epigastric _____

29. Urethrocystitis _____

30. Hypothyroidism _____

31. Traumatology _____

32. Pericardiectomy _____

33. Syndrome _____

34. Hepatorrhaphy _____

35. Megalodactylism _____

36. Nephropexy _____

37. Pneumonomelanosis _____

38. Cerebrovascular _____

39. Chondromalacia _____

40. Amniocentesis _____

41. Inframammary _____

42. Leukocytolysis _____

43. Salpingectomy _____

44. Hemodialysis _____

45. Metastasis _____

46. Cyanopia _____

47. Ophthalmopathy _____

48. Pneumohemothorax _____

49. Otorhinolaryngologist _____

50. Primagravida _____

Answers to Final Self-Test II

1. pendulous, drooping breast
2. nosebleed
3. cessation of menstruation
4. a substance that counteracts (acts against) the effects of a fever
5. a stone (calculus) in the kidney
6. dilatation (stretching) of the small intestine
7. of, or pertaining to, a sudden recurrent onset of a condition (convulsions)
8. hemorrhage within the brain
9. hernia of structures in the skull (cranium)
10. loss of appetite
11. inflammation of the gums and tongue
12. inflammation of the gallbladder
13. painful abdomen
14. spasm (twitching) of an artery
15. condition of hardening of glandular tissue
16. of, or pertaining to, the duodenum and liver
17. examination of the inside of the bronchi
18. paralysis of the iris
19. making a new permanent opening in the trachea
20. webbing or fusion of fingers or toes
21. rupture of a vein
22. condition due to hidden (undescended) testes
23. resembling a blood clot
24. record (picture) of electrical activity in the brain
25. abnormal development of the spinal cord
26. hiccup, hiccough
27. between the ribs
28. of, or pertaining to, area of belly over stomach
29. inflammation of the urethra and bladder
30. condition of insufficient thyroid excretion
31. the study (science) of injuries and their effect on the body
32. excision of tissue around the heart
33. a group of symptoms occurring together
34. suturing (repairing) the liver
35. condition of abnormally large fingers and toes
36. surgical fixation of the kidney in its normal place
37. condition of black lungs, black lung disease
38. of, or pertaining to, the vessels of the brain
39. condition of softened cartilage tissue
40. puncture of the amniotic sac and withdrawing of fluid
41. below the breast
42. destruction of white blood cells
43. surgical removal of the fallopian tube
44. removal of toxic waste products from the blood
45. spreading of a malignant disease to another organ or location
46. blue vision
47. abnormal condition of the eyes
48. air and blood in the chest cavity
49. physician specialist in ear, nose, and voice box diseases
50. a woman pregnant for the first time

Appendix A: Medical Abbreviations

ad libitum (ad. lib.)	As much as wanted; freely
ante cibum (a.c.)	Before meals
bis in die (b.i.d.)	Twice daily
(b.p.)	Blood pressure
cubic centimeter (cc.)	Cubic centimeter(s)
cum (/c)	With
en.	Enema
gram (g.)	Gram or grams
granum (gr.)	Grain or grains
gutta, guttae (gtt.)	Drop or drops
hoc nocte (h.n.)	Tonight
hora somni (h.s.)	At bedtime
l.	Liter(s)
oculus dexter (O.D.)	Right eye
oculus sinister (O.S.)	Left eye
oz.	Ounce
per anum (p.a.)	By, or through, the anus
per os (p.o.)	By, or through, the mouth
post cibum (p.c.)	After meals
pro re nata (p.r.n.)	According to circumstances
quaque die (q.d.)	Every day
quaque hora (q.h.)	Every hour
quater in die (q.i.d.)	Four times daily
signa (sig.)	Let it be labeled
sine (/s)	Without
statim (stat.)	Immediately; at once
suppositoria (suppos.)	Suppository
tabella (tab.)	Tablet
ter in die (t.i.d.)	Three times daily
T.	Temperature

Appendix B: Forming Plurals

The following chart contains information about the formation of plurals from the singular form. Use it to work the frames that follow.

To Form Plurals	
If the singular ending is	**The plural ending is**
a	ae (pronounce ae as ī)
us	i
um	a
ma	mata
on	a
is	es
ix	ices ⎱ The word root is usually built
ex	ices ⎰ from the plural forms of
ax	aces ⎰ words ending in ix, ex, and ax
	(e.g., radix, radic/es,
	radic/otomy, radic/i/form).

bursae
bur′ sī

conjunctivae
kon junk′ tī vē

bacilli
bə sil′ ē

1.
Form the plural of

bursa _____ ;

conjunctiva _____ ;

bacillus _____ .

vertebra
ver′ tə bra

nucleus
noo′ klē us

cornea
kor′ nē ə

2.
Give the singular form of

vertebrae _____ ;

nuclei _____ ;

cornea _____ .

atria
ā′ trē ə

cocci
kok′ sē

ilea
(you pronounce)
il′ ē ə

enema
en′ ə mä

bacterium

ovum
(you pronounce)

cortices
kor′ ti sēz

fibromata
fī brō′ mä tä

protozoa
prō′ to zō′ ə

stigma
stig′ mä

prognosis
prog nō′ sis

spermatozoon
sper mat′ ə zō ən

appendices
(you pronounce)

diagnoses
dī ag nō′ sēz

ganglia
gang′ lē ä

appendic

3.
Form the plural of

atrium _____ ;

coccus _____ ;

ileum _____ .

4.
Give the singular form of

enemata _____ ;

bacteria _____ ;

ova _____ .

5.
Form the pleural of

cortex _____ ;

fibroma _____ ;

protozoon _____ .

6.
Give the singular form of

stigmata _____ ;

prognoses _____ ;

spermatozoa _____ .

7.
Form the plural of

appendix _____ ;

diagnosis _____ ;

ganglion _____ .

8.
Refer to the table. Give the word root that usually refers to

the appendix _____ ;

cortic the cortex _____;

thorac the thorax _____.
(you pronounce)

9.
With this new knowledge, which you found for yourself, build
a word meaning inflammation of the appendix,

appendic/itis
a pen di sī′ tis _____ / _____;
cortic/al pertaining to the cortex,
kor′ ti kəl _____ / _____;
thorac/o/centesis surgical puncture of the thorax,
thor′ ə kō sen tē′ sis _____ / _____ / _____.

10.
Form the plural of

apices apex _____;
fornices fornex _____;
varices varix _____;
sarcomata sarcoma _____;
septa septum _____;
radii radius _____;
maxillae maxilla _____.
(you pronounce)

11.
There are other ways of forming plurals. They apply to only a few
words. When you meet these words and have a question about how
their plural forms are built, consult a medical dictionary.

Index of Words and Word Parts

The following words and word parts are listed by page number.